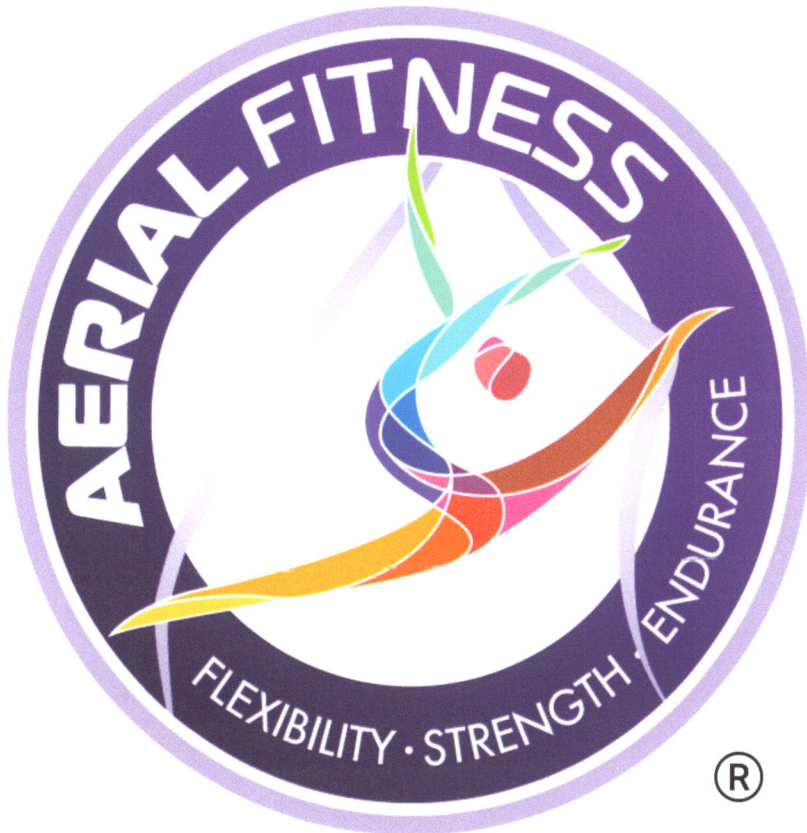

AERIAL FITNESS
A Practical Guide For All Levels

By: Kristi Toguchi
AERIAL FITNESS LLC

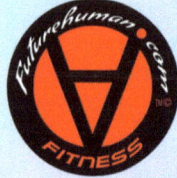

Futurehuman Corporation
1605 John Street
Fort Lee, New Jersey 07024

ISBN: 978-1-953793-06-5 (hc)
ISBN: 978-1-953793-05-8 (sc)
ISBN: 978-1-953793-07-2 (e)

Library of Congress Control Number: 2023915392

Printed in the United States of America
First Printing

Cover Photograph and Design: Beckett Studios
Photography: Richard Faverty
Photography: Shane O'Neal

The exercises and suggestions are not intended as a substitute for consulting with your healthcare provider. In the event you use any of the information in this book for yourself, the author and publisher assume no responsibility for any loss, injury, or damage allegedly arising from any information or suggestion in this book.

Aerial Fitness LLC
www.Aerial-Fitness.net

WELCOME FRIEND

Aerial Fitness was a workout created to fulfill my dream of making my passion for aerial silks accessible to the general public. I want everyone to be able to use aerial silks as a fun and unique way to get healthy and fit. The Aerial Fitness program creates confidence and new body awareness. I believe that it gives you a feeling of power and a feeling of flight by touching the aerial silk. The aerial silk is more than just another fitness tool. It is truly your new fitness partner.

Kristi Toguchi

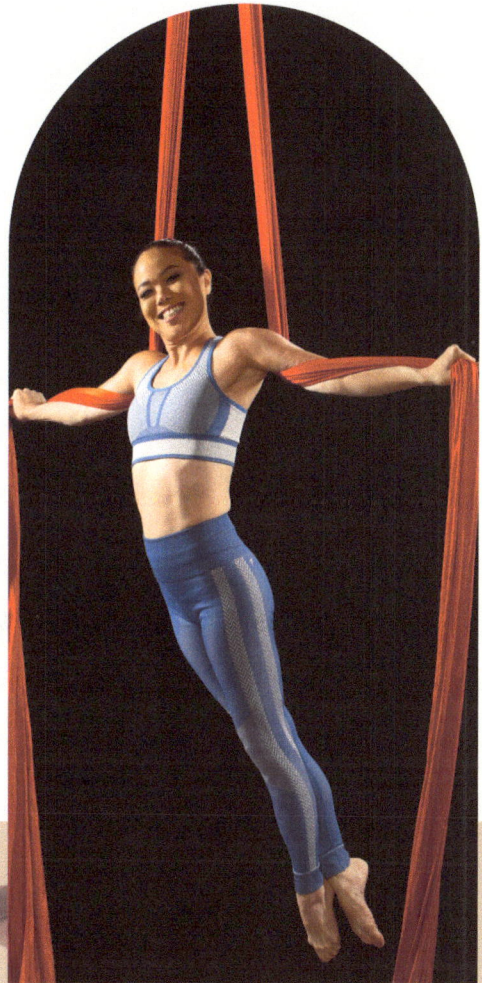

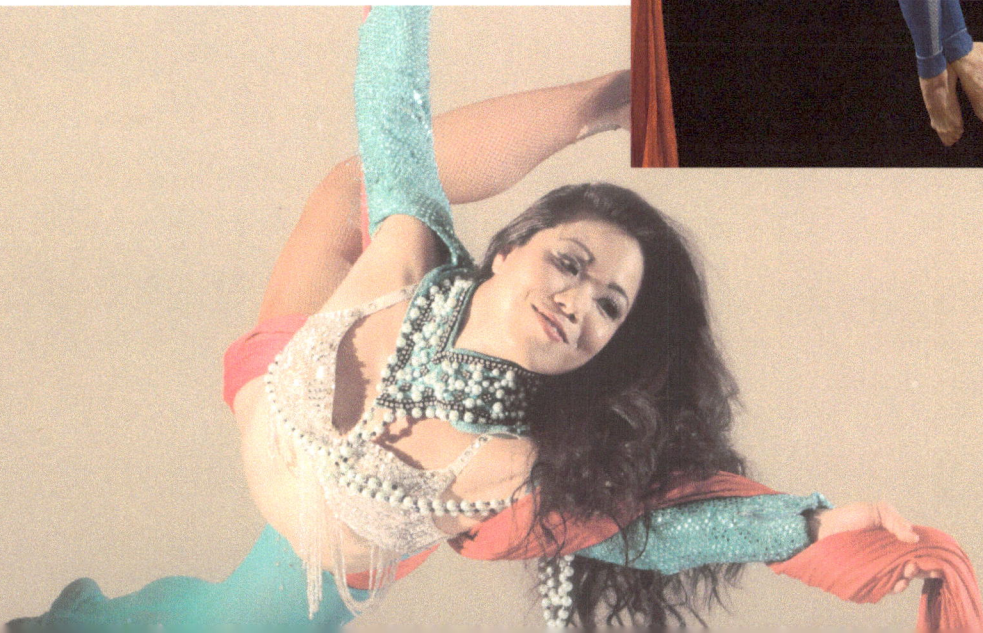

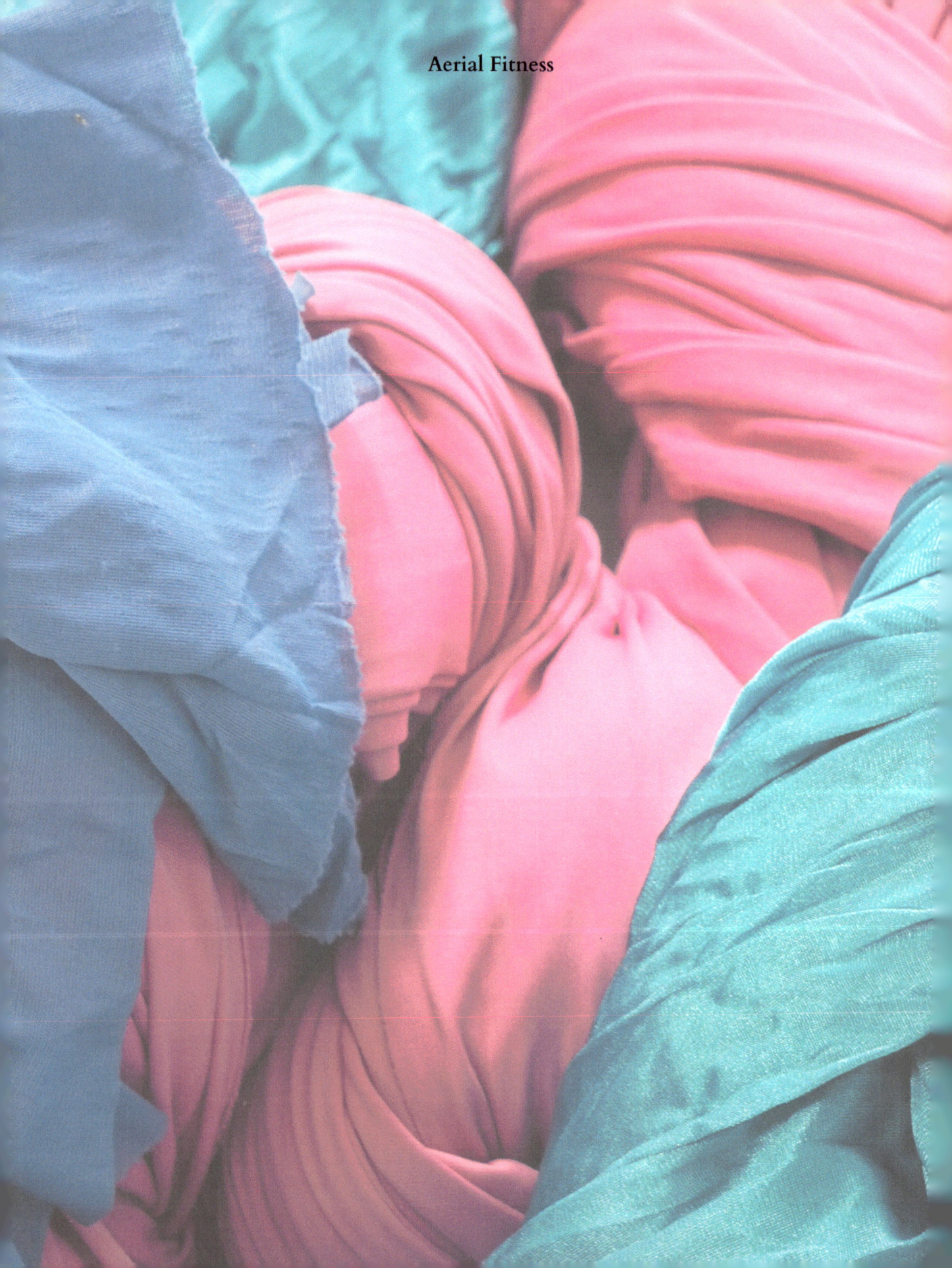

✦

KRISTI TOGUCHI

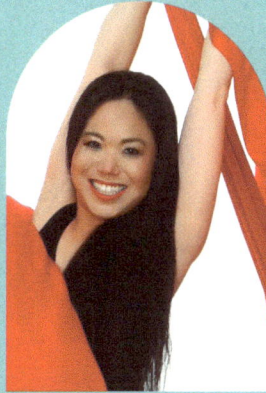

Kristi Toguchi is the founder of Aerial Fitness®, co-founder of Futurehuman®, and a world-class entertainer and coach. Kristi has been featured by more than 100 media outlets, including NBC, Fox, SyFy, Discovery, Travel Channel, HGTV, Amazon Studios, Sony, Muscle & Fitness Magazine, GQ, Golf Magazine, and Thomas Cook Travel Magazine. She was also the resident aerialist at the world-famous Tao Night Club in Las Vegas, Nevada.

Kristi has over 25 years of teaching experience, specializing in aerial acrobatics, contortion, dance, and magic. She has taught students worldwide, and she is the owner of Aerial Fitness® School (www.AerialFitness.us) in Las Vegas. Her students have attended the prestigious Ecole National Circus School. Many of them have gone on to have successful careers performing in international venues, including the Olympics, cruise lines, television, corporate events, and more.

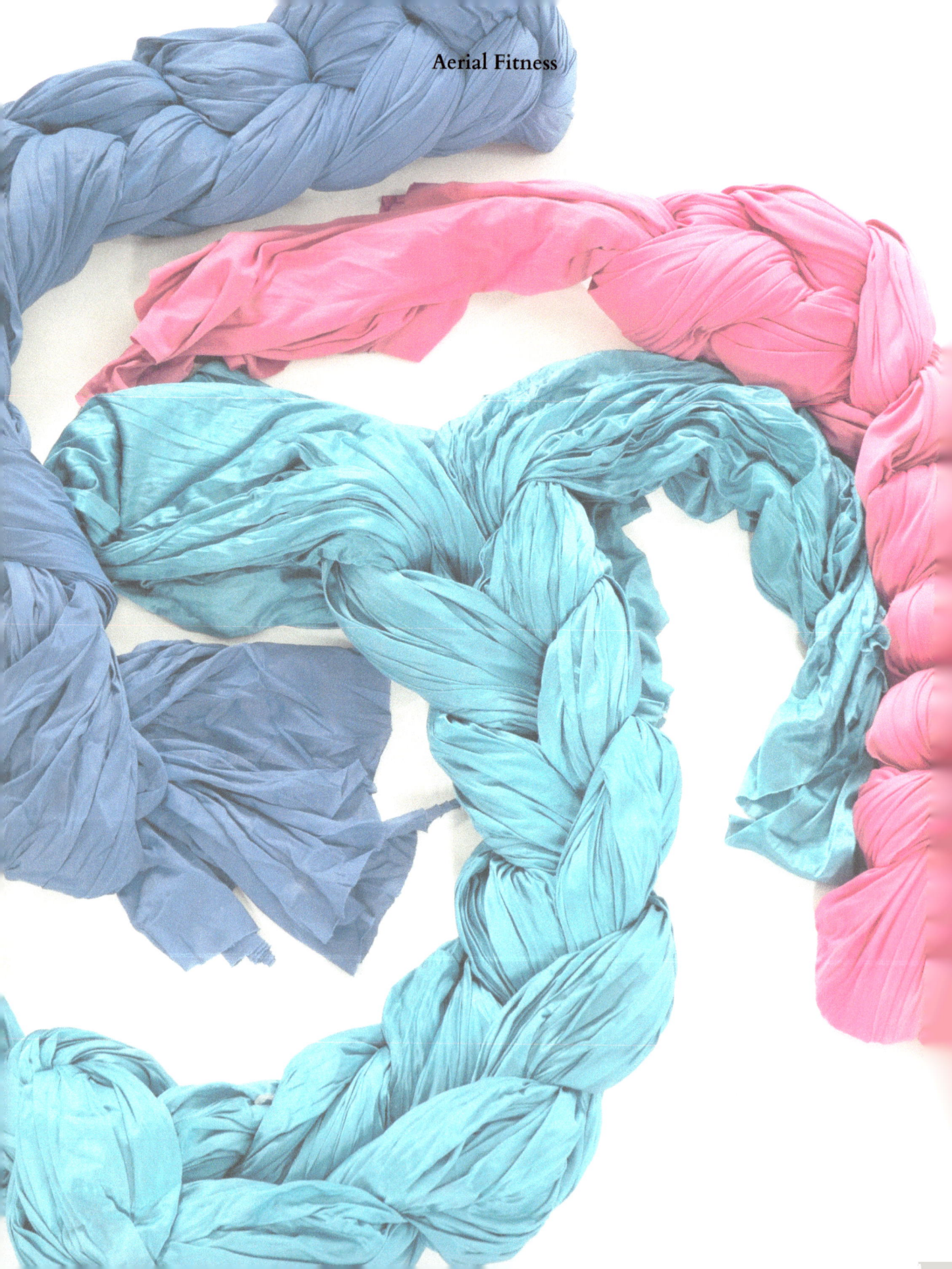

DISCLAIMER

PROCEED AT YOUR OWN RISK

Aerial Fitness was written with the belief that you can build a smart and safe Aerial Fitness program at home. However, if you have any concerns about the Aerial Fitness exercise's impact on your physical health, please consult a physician before attempting any of the exercises in this book. Ensure your equipment is set up correctly and tested before proceeding to do any Aerial Fitness exercises in this book. The exercises in this book are intended to be performed on the ground or close to the ground. Professional aerialists train for years to accomplish amazing feats high above the sky. Please do not attempt these dangerous acts without proper aerial instruction from a professional coach. The publisher and author are not liable for any complications, injuries, loss, or medical problems arising from or in connection with using this book.

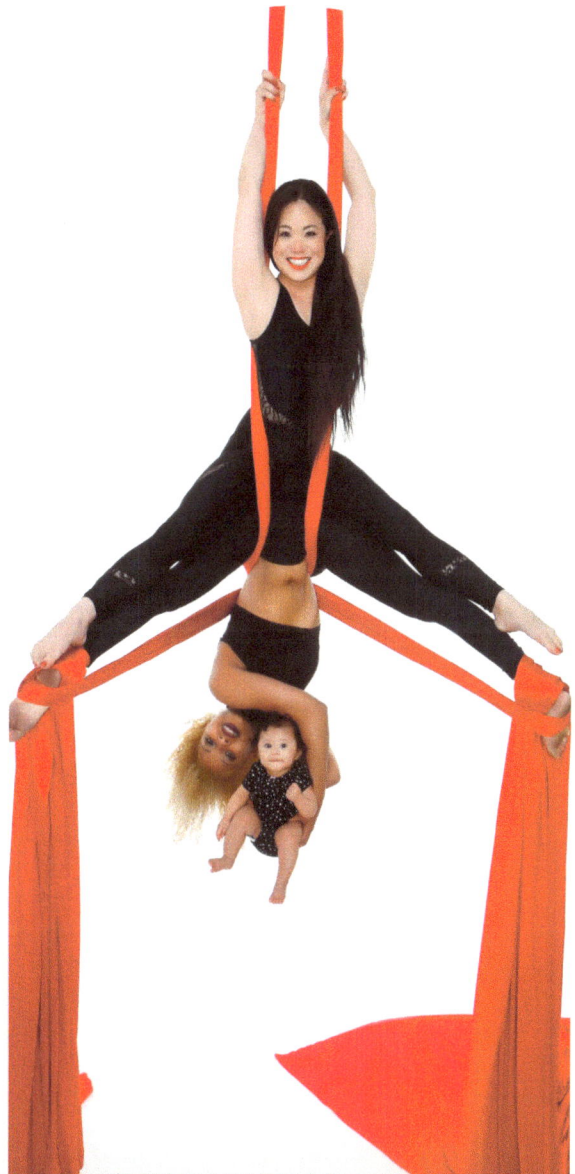

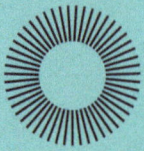

TABLE OF CONTENTS

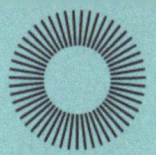

TABLE OF CONTENTS

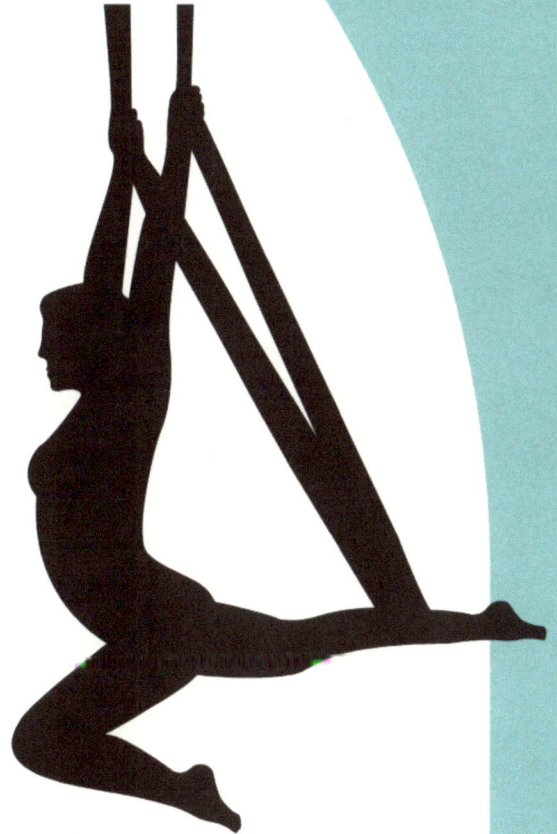

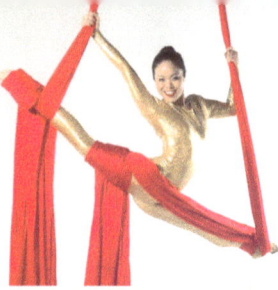

INTRODUCTION

Aerial Fitness will focus on building your upper body, core strength, and overall flexibility. You will learn exercises moving your body off the ground and into the air. This exercise program is a full-body workout that will emphasize building technique and proper alignment. You will use the aerial silk to condition your body by doing bodyweight exercises and stretches while being attached to the aerial silk.

Additionally, you will learn the foundations of Aerial Fitness, including climbing, inversions, and other fundamental movements that will help you build comfort and safety awareness with the equipment. Aerial Fitness is a great workout to get into shape, stay in shape, or prepare for other aerial acrobatic classes (aerial silk, aerial hoop, trapeze, etc.).

The Aerial Fitness book is a complete training program and guide for operating a safe, mindful, and successful Aerial Fitness practice.

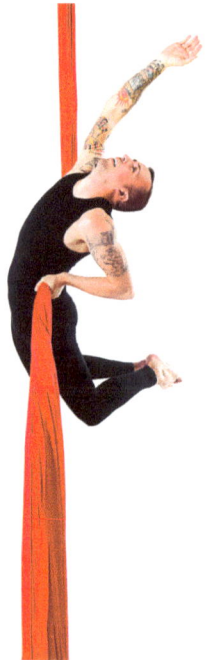

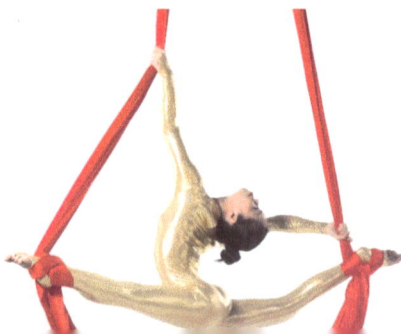

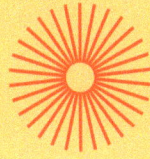

KEY ELEMENTS OF AERIAL FITNESS

- building a foundation of strong core muscles
- building a relationship with your apparatus–the aerial silk
- focusing on the core muscles to stabilize your body in the air
- controlling your movements to build strength and precision
- finding your breath through the movement
- improving your mind–body connection
- understanding your body awareness on a 360° dimension
- understanding aerial safety and proper body mechanics
- developing focus and concentration
- improving your memory
- utilizing proper techniques to prevent injury

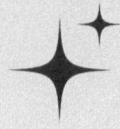

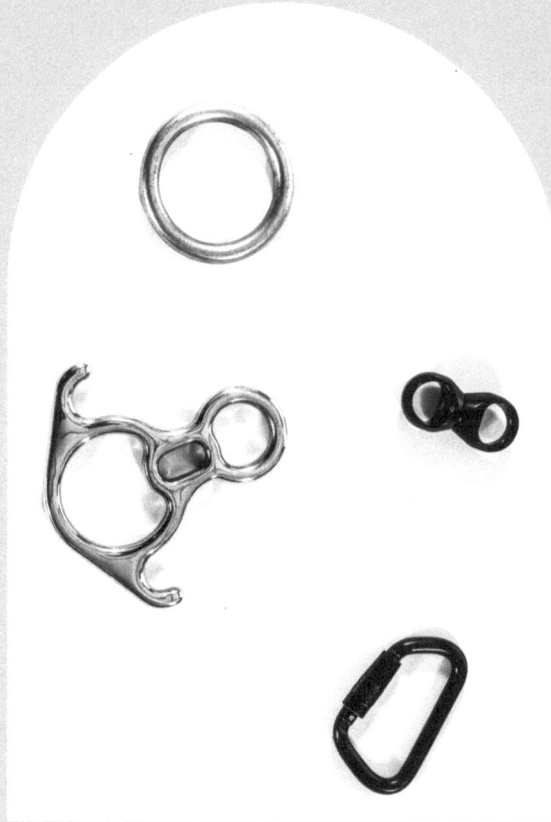

AERIAL FITNESS EQUIPMENT

The exercises in this book are intended for those who have access to professional aerial silk rigging. Some movements in this book do not require any equipment; however, most exercises will be done with the aerial silk apparatus. You can purchase Aerial Fitness equipment from a company that specializes in creating aerial equipment. There is a list of resources at the end of this book. To accomplish the exercises in this book, you will need the minimum requirement of an aerial fabric and proper rigging.

Essential equipment includes a steel figure 8 or an "O" Ring, a locking carabiner (double or triple lock preferred for extra safety), a thick mat or crash pad, and an aerial silk fabric (24 ft-60 ft in length, measures 12 ft-30 ft when rigged). Additional recommended equipment includes another carabiner and a swivel. Some also like to use rosin to help with grip on the fabric.

Even though you purchase all of the above equipment, you will still need a safe way to rig your aerial silk before you can begin your Aerial Fitness workout. The easiest solution is to go to your local park and find a monkey bar or pull-up bar you can use to attach the fabric. It is even possible to do many of the exercises with an at-home pull-up bar that is safely installed. These rigging options will be discussed in detail.

The safest solution is to find a studio that can accommodate your aerial silk rigging. Luckily, with the popularity of aerial yoga, *American Ninja Warrior*, and other circus workouts, studios with accommodations are very common in most cities. If you would like to practice your Aerial Fitness technique at home, we recommend purchasing a professional aerial rigging from a reputable company or hiring a professional rigger. Altering the infrastructure of your living quarters without professional help could have catastrophic results. A mat is also needed anytime you practice Aerial Fitness.

Aerial Fitness equipment can be purchased at various online retailers, including rigging companies, circus equipment companies, sports equipment companies, and even your local fabric store.

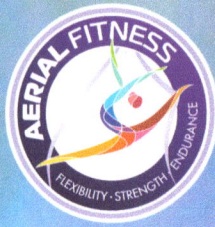

PRO TIP:

ALWAYS REMEMBER TO INSPECT YOUR RIGGING. REMOVE ALL YOUR RIGGING FROM THEIR ATTACHMENTS (INCLUDING THE AERIAL SILK FROM THE O-RING, BAR, OR FIGURE-8) TO MAKE SURE THEY ARE NOT COMPROMISED

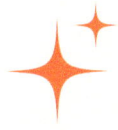

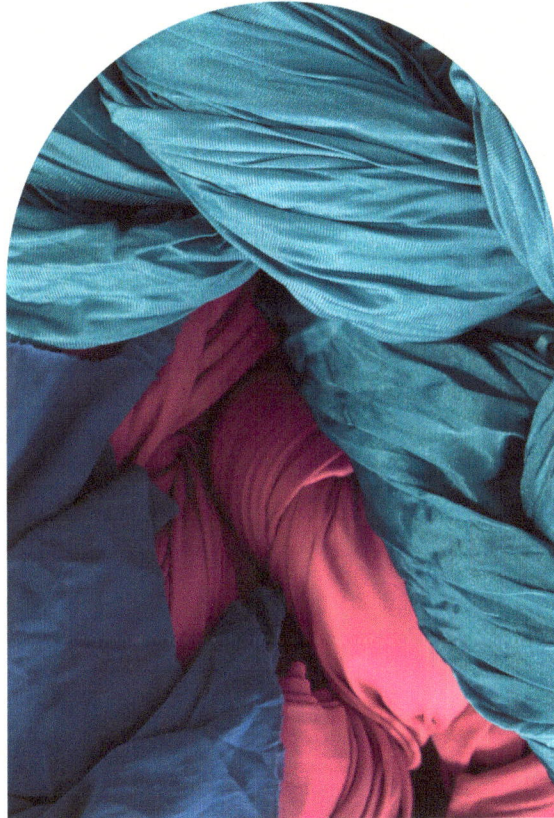

AERIAL FITNESS

FABRIC SELECTION

Aerial silk fabric can be most commonly purchased online at independent retailers and is available in many colors, lengths, and stretch levels. Selecting the type of material you use for your Aerial Fitness workout is a personal decision, dependent on your personal preference, rigging options, body size, and level of experience.

Many silk vendors will categorize the aerial fabric into a few categories: low-stretch, medium-stretch, high-stretch, tricot, polyester interlock, and widths.

The fabric must come in one continuous bolt for the material's integrity to remain safe and secure. It cannot be sewn together.

The low-stretch fabric is more static and generally more comfortable to climb and manipulate for beginners.

The materials that come in a smaller width are more manageable for children.

The tricot fabric tends to be more of a low to medium-stretch material with more options for wider widths, while the polyester interlock fabric is a more medium to high-stretch fabric that tends to have many more color options.

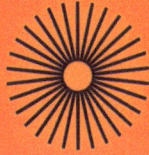

AERIAL SILK MAINTENANCE

It is essential to take care of your aerial silk. You should inspect your fabric by opening the material up and looking for any holes and runs. You should pay particular attention to parts of the material attached to any rigging. Over time, the fabric's natural wear and tear will happen, and you will notice the fabric will look and feel different. The material will weaken, especially where it is attached to any rigging or equipment. Observe this part of the fabric. It should be replaced when it starts to become thin, or if you see any large runs or holes in your material.

For hygiene purposes, you may wash the aerial fabric. You may want to get your material professionally cleaned. If you have a large washer, you can also do it yourself.

Monitor and replace the rigging equipment as recommended by the manufacturing company. You can look for cracks or deformities in your equipment to indicate that your rigging is about to fail. You may also hear different clicks or noises that could demonstrate the integrity of the equipment.

When not in use, many people will use a daisy chain technique to shorten the fabric's length to conveniently store the aerial silk. To create the Aerial Silk Daisy Chain, you will use the same method you would for a crochet chain.

AERIAL SILK DAISY CHAIN

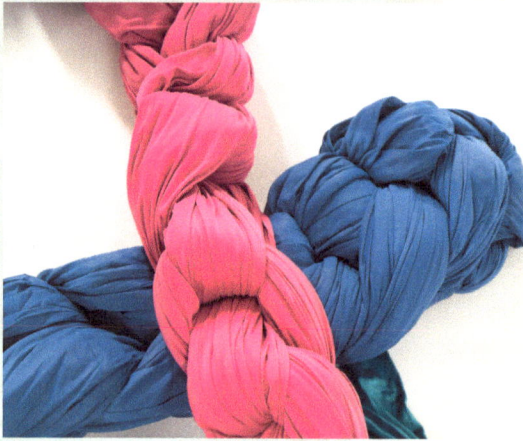

The technique of creating a daisy chain with the aerial silk is very similar to creating a crochet daisy chain, except your arm and hands replace the crochet needle.

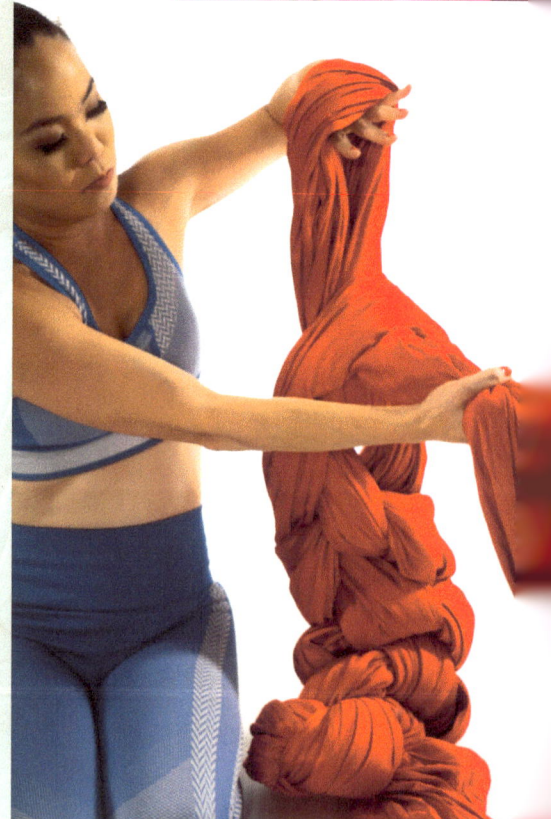

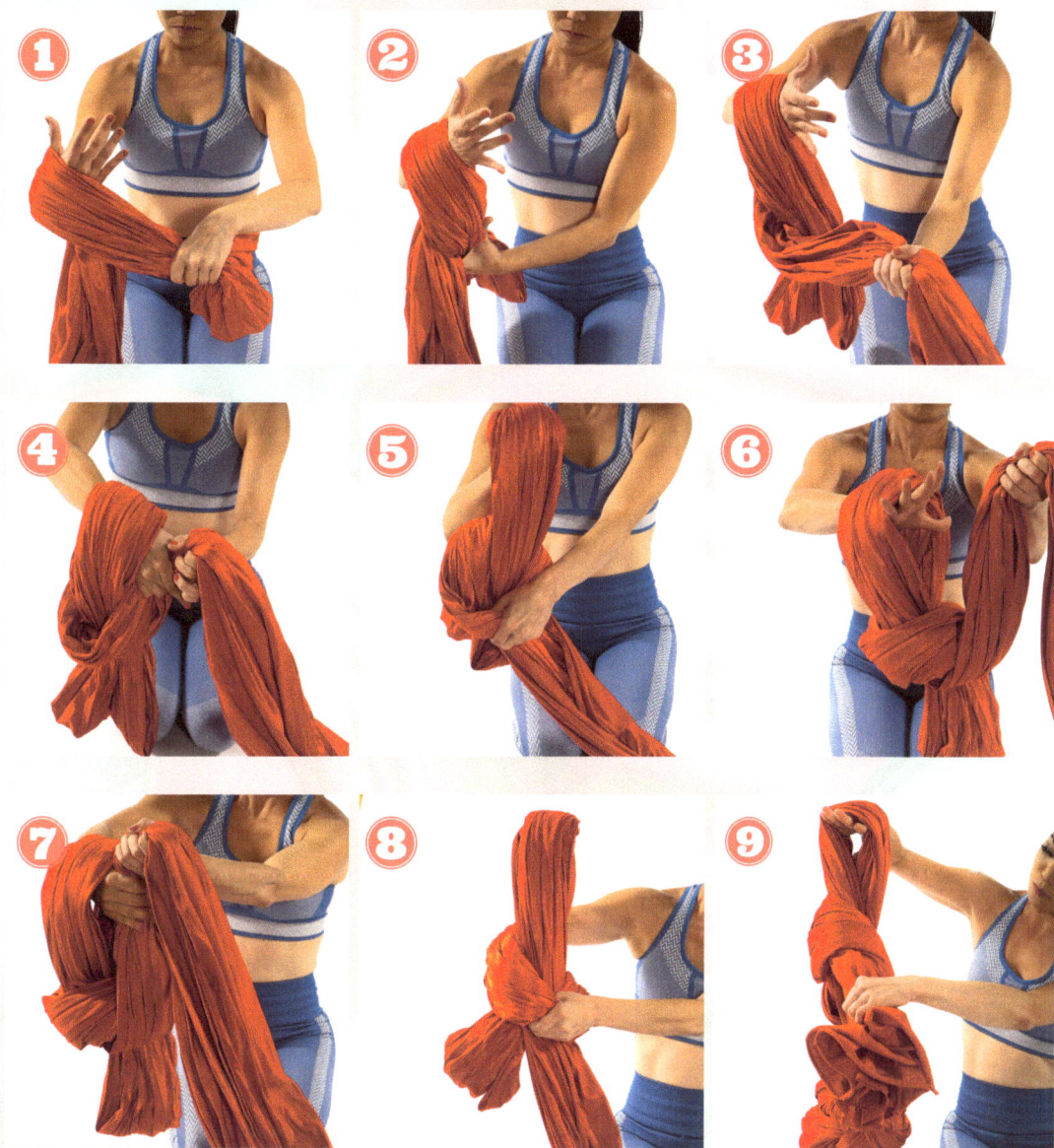

First, grab the two silks together and wrap them around one wrist as you would do to make a hand knot. With the other hand, pick up the fabric dangling under the bound hand and bring it over your wrist from your thumb to your pinky finger, so it creates an "X" over the top of your wrist. Grip the fabric above your hand with the other hand. Now, pull the material through the hole that has been created. Finally, cinch the knot to secure it. The more slack you have when you grab the fabric (i.e., the closer you hold to the tail end of the fabric), the larger the hole is created, making it easier for the fabric to pass through.

AERIAL FITNESS

SIMPLE RIGGING METHODS

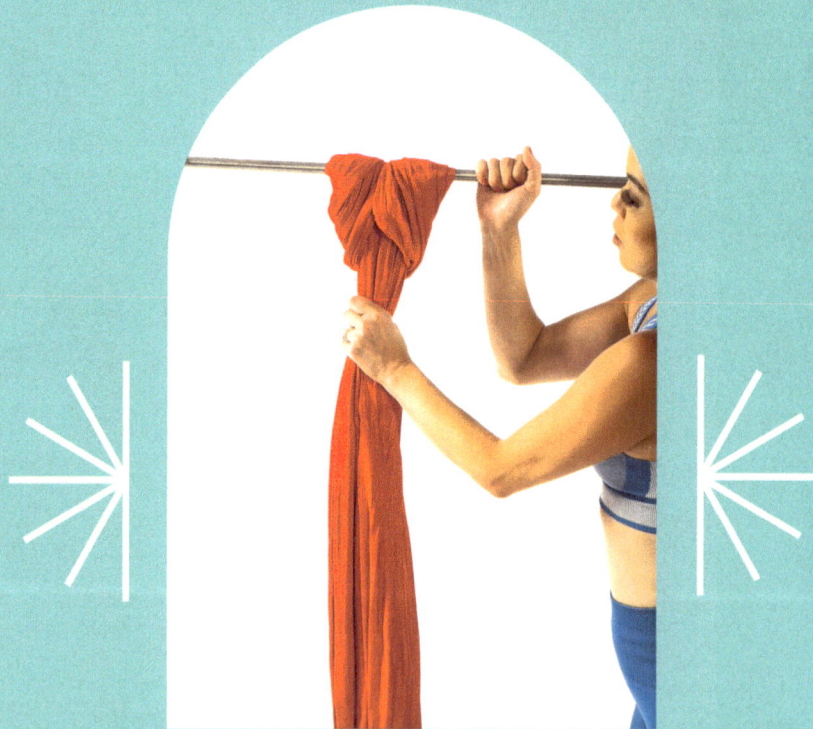

We highly recommend professional rigging. However, we understand that the costs of equipment may be too much for many people. Safety should be the top priority in any aerial training program regardless of how high anyone is off the ground. The Aerial Fitness program will allow access to practice without having a high clearance.

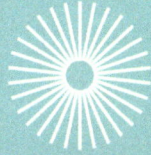

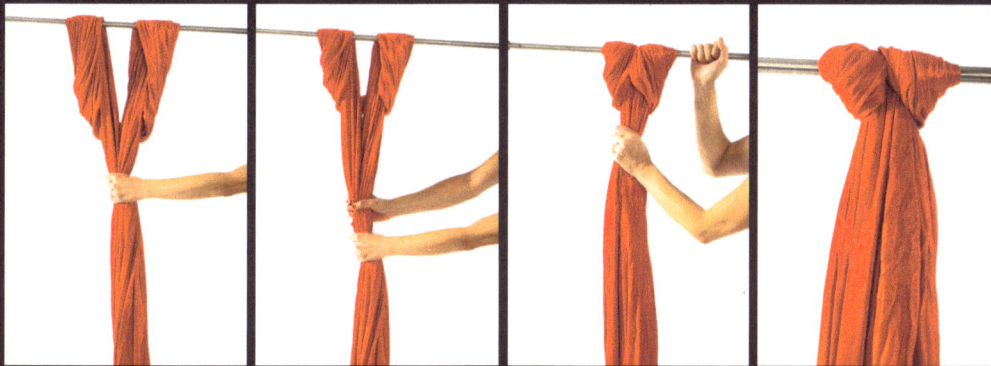

Most exercises can be accomplished with simple at-home rigging. First, purchase the preferred pull-up bar and safely install it according to the manufacturer's guidelines. Test the pull-up bar with the manufacturer's recommended exercises. Make sure all rigging has structural integrity and can manage the pounds of pressure and weight that can be exerted by you. Purchase about 6–9 yards of aerial silk fabric (depending on the height you would like to set up your rigging at). Affix the material by folding the fabric in half to tie a girth hitch knot onto the pull-up bar.

The girth hitch knot method may also be applied at many local parks and gyms equipped with pull-up or monkey bars.

Always inspect the fabric before every use to ensure there are no runs, tears, or holes in the material.

AERIAL FITNESS

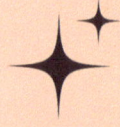

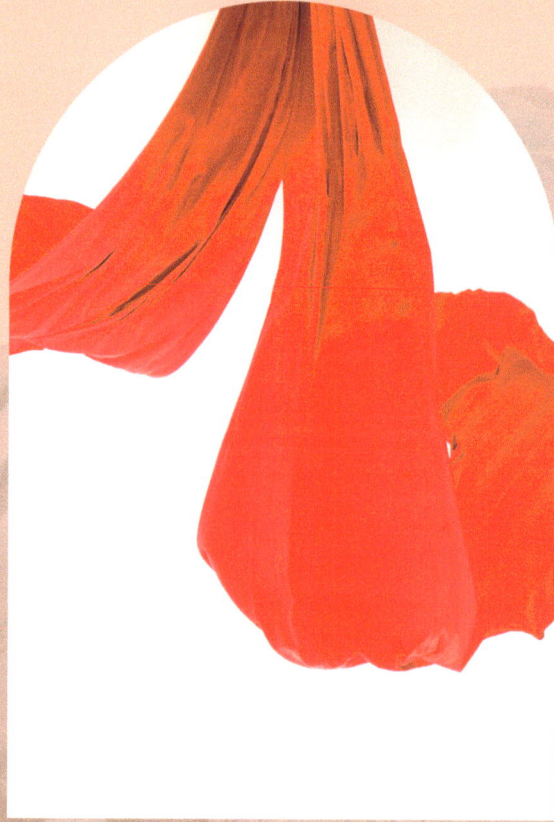

HISTORY OF AERIAL SILKS

Aerial Fitness

The exact origin of the art of aerial silk or aerial tissu is a hearsay tale. The story began in 1959 when a young French circus school student was challenged to make a new circus act to present. It is rumored that the student, who trained in corde lisse (an aerial rope apparatus), presented the first modern aerial silk act with a long piece of fabric he purchased at a local market. Although this first aerial silk act's creator remains a mystery, an article was published in a local newspaper to document the event.

Unfortunately, there is no other documentation of the art until January 1995. Under the creation of André Simard, Isabelle Vaudelle presented the first aerial silk act to the public at the Festival Mondial du Cirque de Demain, which was filmed at the Cirque d'Hiver–Bouglione.

In 1998, the aerial silks became a global phenomenon as Isabelle Vaudelle and Isabelle Chasse performed their aerial silk act in Cirque Du Soleil's Quidam. Many acrobats worldwide began to experiment with aerial silk or aerial tissu, and new methods and creations began to happen all the time. Before the existence of aerial silks, aerialists performed the corde lisse or Spanish web act. Many of the movements and tricks on the ropes easily transitioned on to the aerial silks.

Along with the innovation of new tricks on the aerial silks came new apparatus. Now we have an aerial hammock, aerial net, aerial chain, and aerial slings, and the list will continue to grow as aerial acrobatics' popularity grows. Today you can see aerial performances in many venues, and aerial artists continue to push the boundaries of what we once thought was possible.

Aerial Fitness
(ˈer-ē-əl fit-ness)

the condition of getting physically fit and healthy existing, happening, or operating in the air

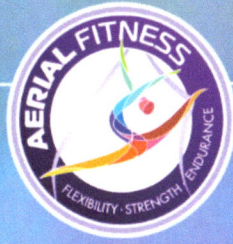

Want to improve your flexibility training? This will help...

✓ Remember to breathe

✓ Use props that can assist you in stretching

✓ Use a yoga mat to help you with your alignment in positions

AERIAL FITNESS

WARM-UP & COOL-DOWN

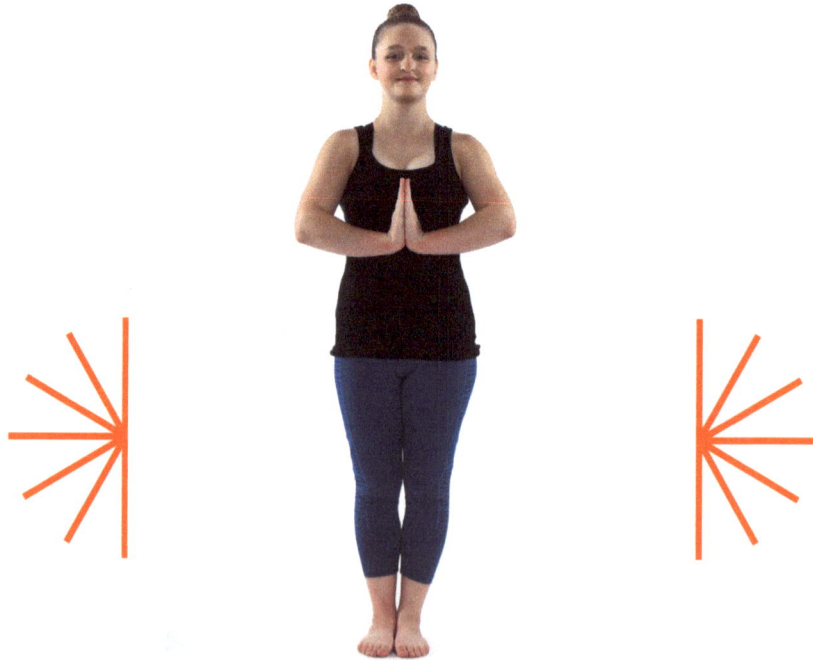

Warming up and cooling down your body is an essential part of the Aerial Fitness program.

Warming up and cooling down your body is a great pre and post-care routine for your training program. A proper warm-up will help you keep your body safe and prevent injury by increasing the temperature and supplying oxygen to your muscles. This will allow your body to be the most strong and most flexible during your training session.

Cooling down your body is also extremely important to add to your routine to help regulate your blood flow when you have completed your training. Post-workout stretches can help you increase your range of motion and delay muscle fatigue.

Warm-Up Routine

- **NECK: HEAD CIRCLES-** To begin, place your right ear to your right shoulder, then place your chin on your chest, then place your left ear to your left shoulder, continue the circle to look up to the sky, and continue to place your right ear on your right shoulder. Continue this pattern for 5-10 rotations, then rotate in the other direction.

- **SHOULDERS: ARM CIRCLES-** To begin, stand up tall. Place your legs together, feet together, and pull your navel into your spine. Slowly rotate your arms in a circular motion from front to back or clockwise with straight arms. Imagine drawing a large circle with the fingertips of each hand. Do 1 set of 10. Repeat and rotate your arms in a circular motion from back to front or counterclockwise with straight arms. Do 1 set of 10. Repeat as necessary.

- **HANDS & WRIST: WRIST EXTENSION DOWN-** To begin, stand up tall. Glue your legs together, feet together, and pull your navel into your spine. Extend your arm in front of your body, parallel to the ground palm face up. Pull your fingertips down with the opposite hand and flex at the wrist until you feel a stretch. Hold for 20-30 seconds. Repeat on the other side.

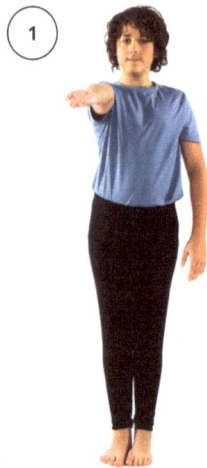

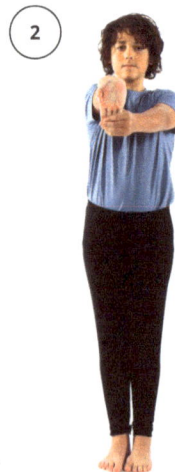

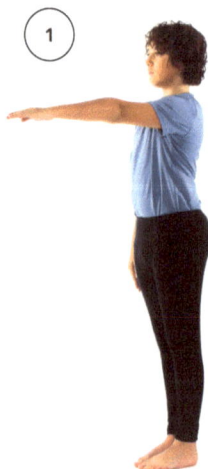

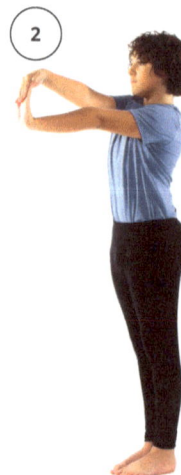

- **WRIST EXTENSION UP-** Extend your arm in front of your body, parallel to the ground palm face down. Pull your fingertips up with the opposite hand and flex at the wrist until you feel a stretch. Hold for 20-30 seconds. Repeat on the other side.

- **ARMS & WRIST: KNEELING WRIST EXTENSION–** Kneel on the ground with your legs and feet glued together. Place your arms shoulder-width apart. Place your palms on the ground with your shoulders stacked over your wrists and fingers pointing toward the knees. Slowly sit until the desired stretch is felt. Hold the stretch for 20–30 seconds. Repeat with the top of the hand on the ground.

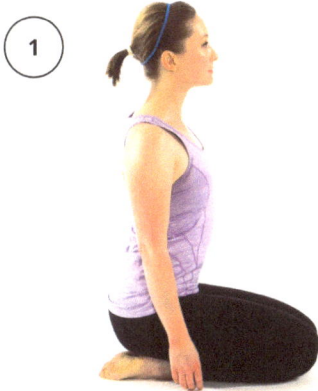

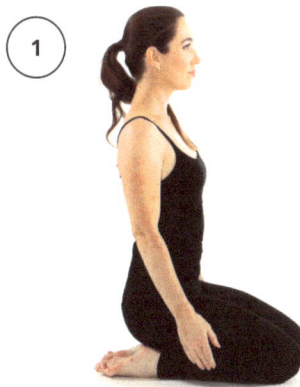

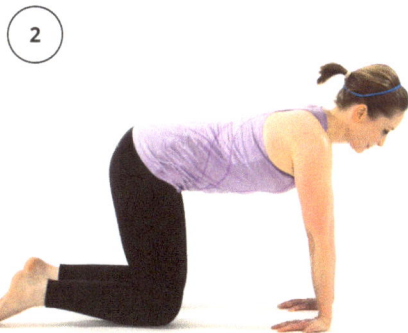

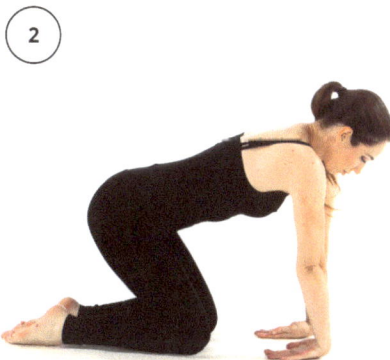

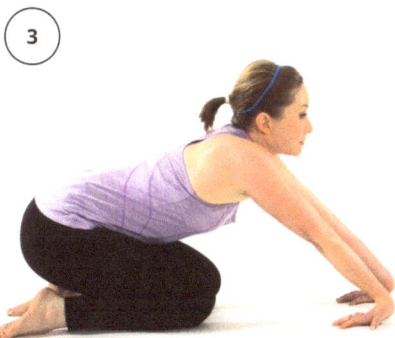

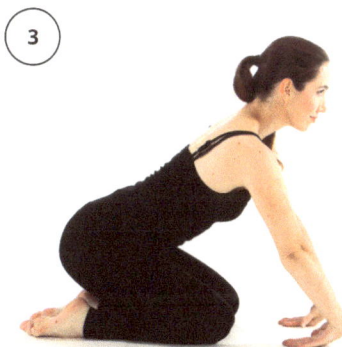

- **WRIST FLEXORS: PRAYER STRETCH-** To begin, stand up tall. Glue your legs together, feet together, and pull your navel into your spine. Place palms together in front of the heart in a prayer position. Rotate your hands and point your fingers toward your neck. Push your hands together and slowly lower them away from the body until the wrists separate. Hold the stretch for 20-30 seconds.

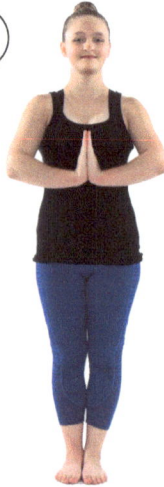 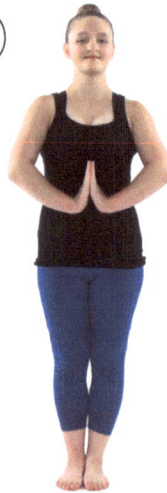 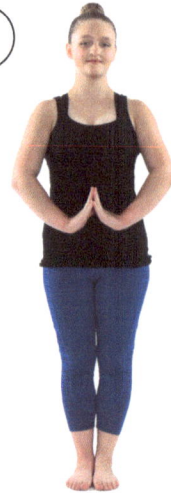

- **BICEPS: BICEP STRETCH-** Fold your right arm across your body parallel to the ground and pull your right shoulder down. With your left shoulder down, push your arm into your body to increase the stretch. Hold the position and turn your head to the left and hold for 20 seconds, then turn your head to the right and hold for 20 seconds. Repeat on the other side.

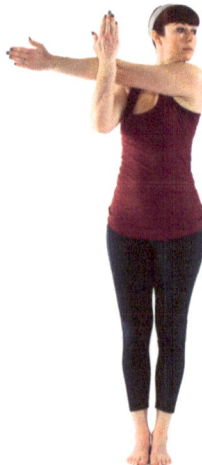

- **TRICEPS: TRICEP STRETCH–** Start with your arms to the side of your body. Lift both arms straight into the air, bend the right elbow, and place your hand palm face down behind the center of your head or neck. From this position, use the opposite arm to push your elbow down toward the center of your spine. Hold for 10-20 seconds. Repeat on the other side.

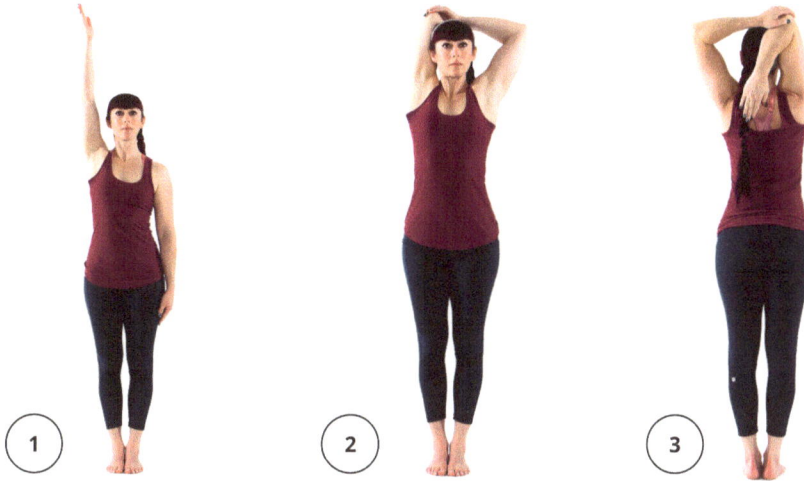

- **CHEST: PECTORAL STRETCH–** To begin, stand up tall with your feet about hip-width apart or wider. Pull your navel into your spine. Clasp your hands together behind your back with your fingers pointing down and wrists apart. Slowly lift your arms until you feel your desired stretch. Hold for 20-30 seconds. For a deeper stretch, repeat with your palms together.

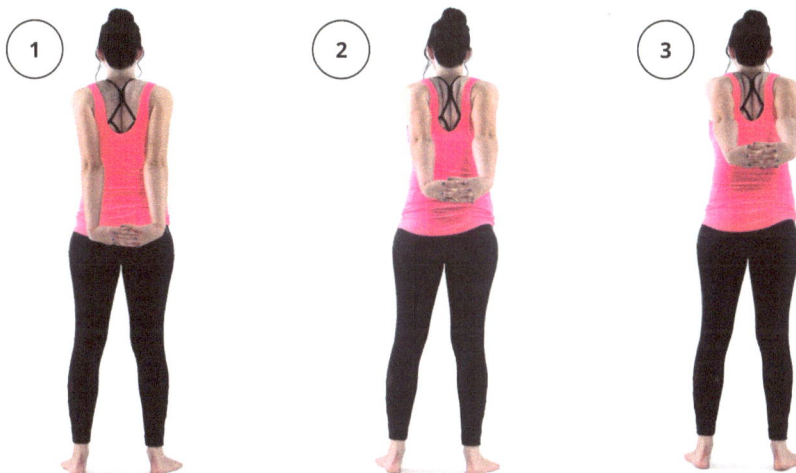

- **ARMS & SHOULDERS: UPPER ARM STRETCH-** To begin, sit on the floor with knees bent and feet on the ground about hip-width apart. Lean back and place your hands close together with your palms down behind your body with fingers pointing away from the body. Slowly move hands away from the body equally until a stretch is felt. Hold for 20-30 seconds.

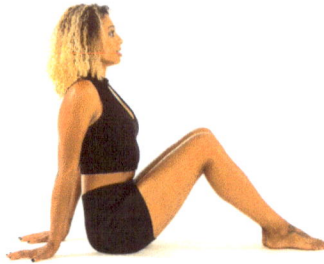

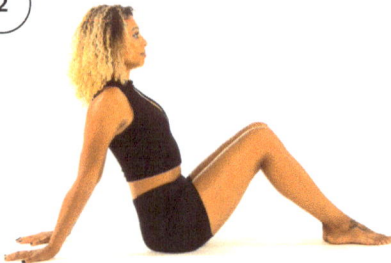

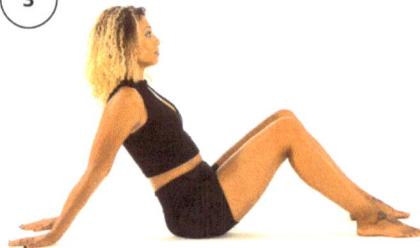

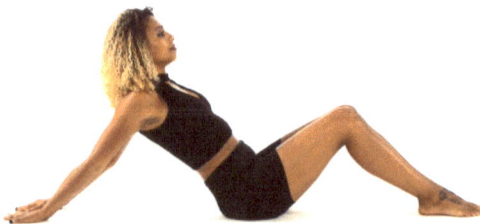

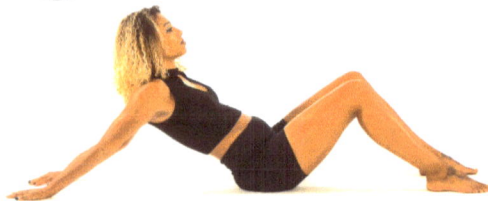

- **HIPS: HIP CIRCLES-** Place your hands on your hips. Push your pelvis forward to feel a stretch in your psoas. Rotate your pelvis in a circular motion to the right hip, then rotate your pelvis in a circular motion to the back pushing your glutes out and bending in your lower back to create a stretch in your lower back. Continue to rotate your pelvis in a circular motion to your left hip. Repeat 5-10 times, then repeat to the other side.

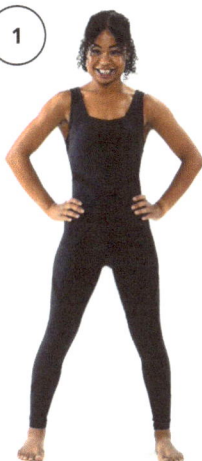 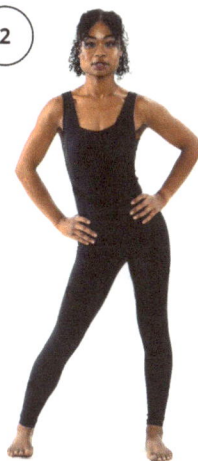

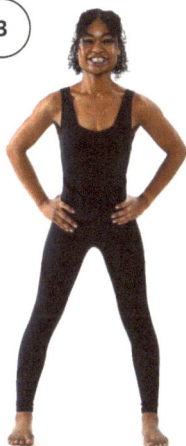 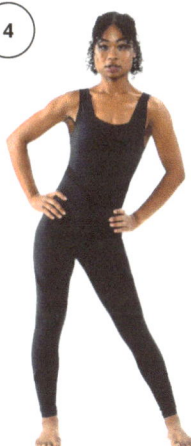

- **HIPS & SHOULDER: 2nd POSITION PECTORAL STRETCH–** Place your legs more than hip-width apart with your toes pointing to the side. Bend your knees and drop your hips so they are parallel to the ground placing your knees over your toes at a 90° angle. Sink your left shoulder to your right knee and hold for 10 seconds. Repeat on the other side.

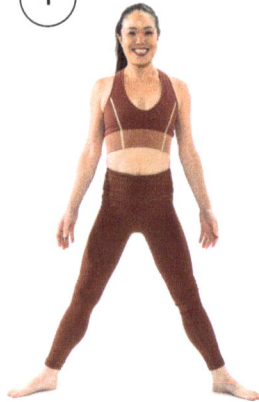

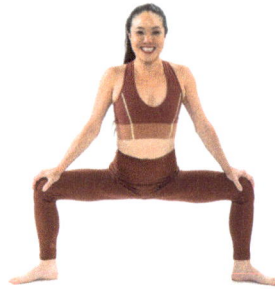

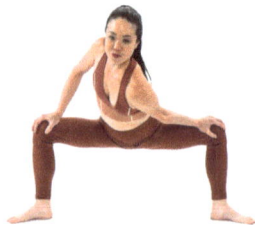

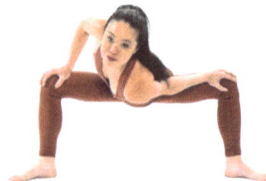

- **HAMSTRING: FORWARD BEND-** Stand with your feet and legs glued together. Pull your chin into your chest, and from the crown of your head start to roll down in a forward bend one vertebrae at a time. Try to place your hands on the ground with your energy moving forward to your toes. Hold each stretch for 10-20 seconds.

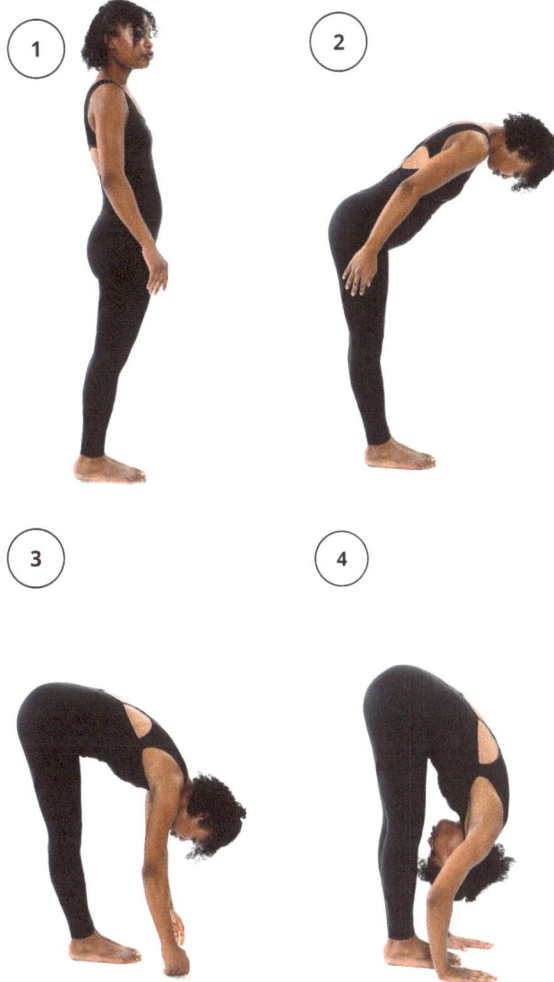

- **HAMSTRING: STRADDLE SPLIT LUNGE-** Stand with your feet and legs glued together. Turn your hips, legs, and feet open like a window in a "V" position or Ballet 1st Position. Step your right leg out in the same line into a deep lunge keeping your knee over your ankle at a 90° angle. Place your hands on the ground in front of your body. Flex your left foot, point your knees and toes up to the sky, and hold for 10-20 seconds. Then point your foot and hold for 10-20 seconds. Repeat on the other side.

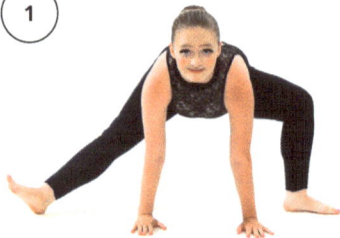
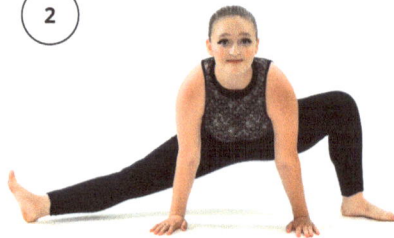

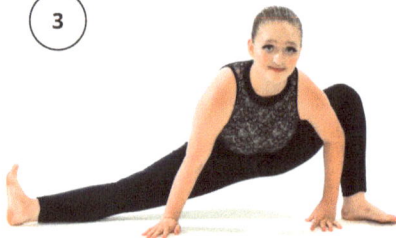
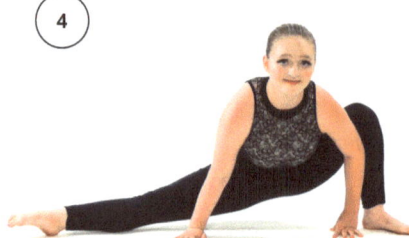

**PRO TIP: WHEN IN A DEEP LUNGE USE THE
SAME ARM AS YOUR LEG TO HELP PUSH THE
KNEE BACK TO DEEPEN YOUR STRETCH**

- **HAMSTRINGS & HIP FLEXORS: STRADDLE/CENTER SPLITS-** From a Butterfly position, extend your legs to a comfortable Center Splits position. Sit up tall on your sit bones and hold for 20-30 seconds.

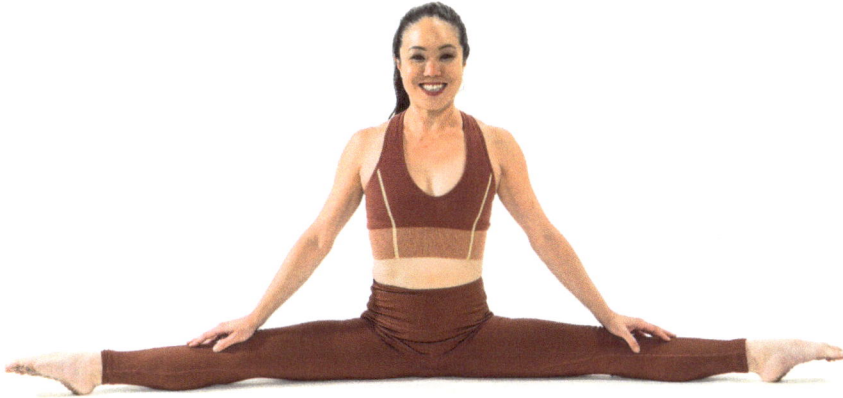

- **HAMSTRING: STRADDLE SPLIT SIDE STRETCH-** Once in your Straddle Split position, shoot your right fingertips to your left leg in front of your body with the top of your arm on the ground with your right palm facing up. Extend your left arm over your head and bend toward your right leg. Be sure to open your left (or top) shoulder down and back. Hold for 10 seconds and repeat on the other side.

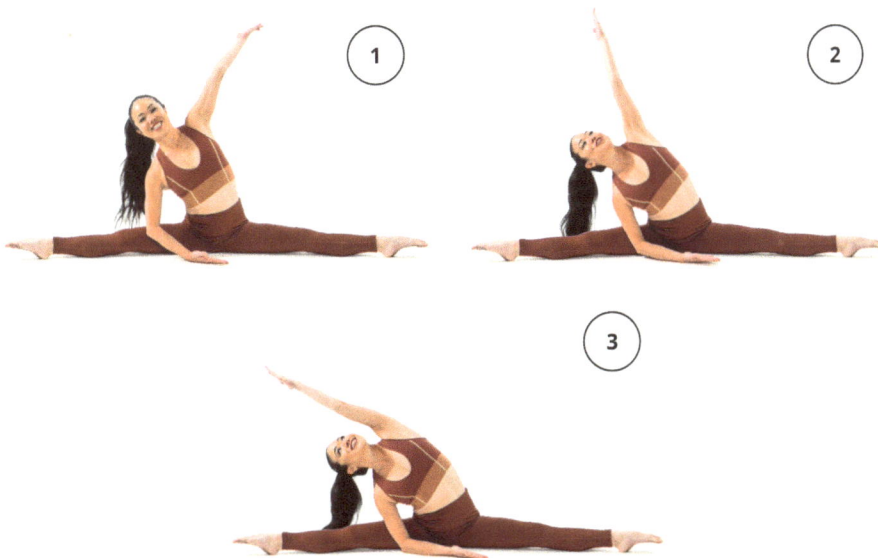

- **HAMSTRING: STRADDLE SPLIT PANCAKE-** From a Straddle Split position, reach your hands forward one at a time. Try to flatten your back from the base of your spine. When you reach your maximum stretch, hold for 20-30 seconds.

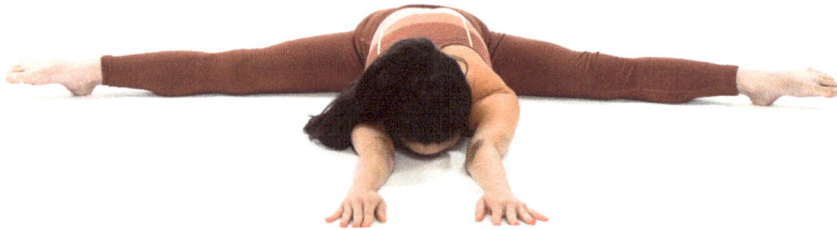

- **HIP FLEXORS: SIDE SPLIT LUNGE-** Stand with your feet and legs glued together. Step your right leg back into a deep lunge with your hands beside your body. Sink your psoas into the ground keeping your back leg straight with your heel up and your front leg at a 90° angle with your knee over your ankle bone. Hold for 10-20 seconds. Repeat on the other side. For more of a challenge, try to sit up tall once in your deep lunge.

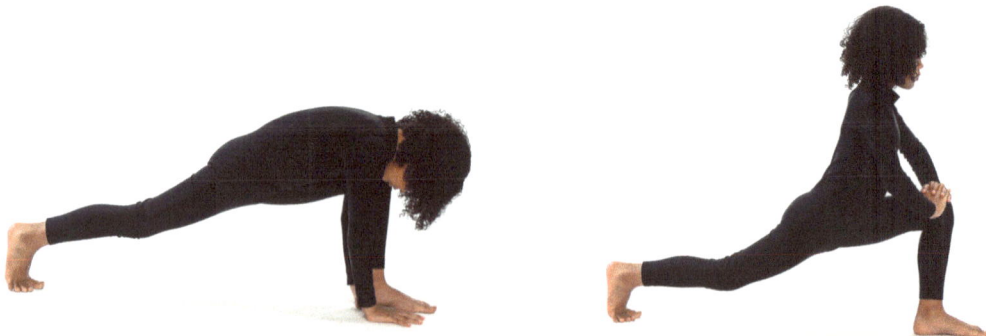

- **HAMSTRINGS & QUADRICEPS: TRIANGLE STRETCH-** From your Side Split Lunge position, and step your back foot in 1-2 feet to make a triangle position. Pull your back hip down and shift your weight forward to square your hips off. Hold for 10-20 seconds.

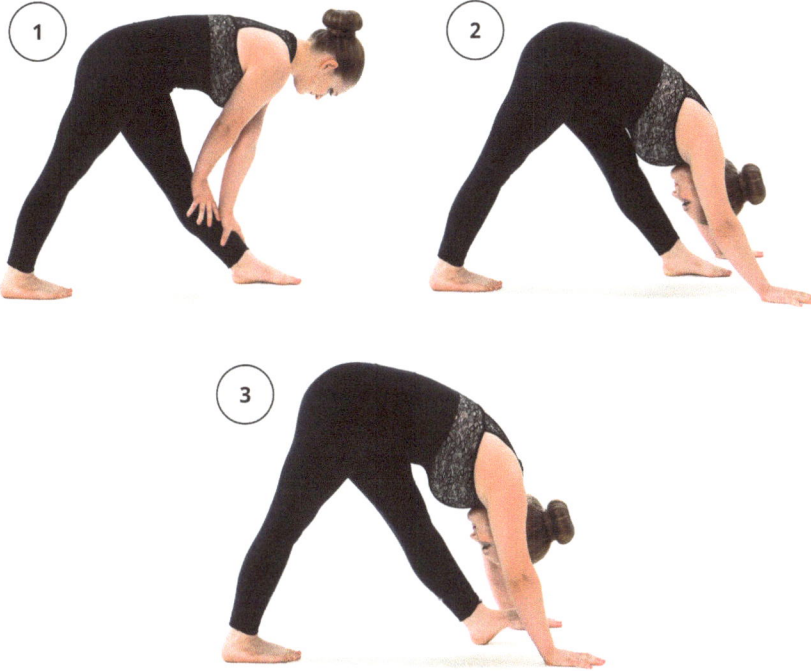

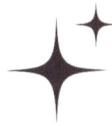

**PRO TIP: FLEX YOUR FRONT FOOT AND
LENGTHEN BEHIND YOUR KNEES
FOR A DEEPER STRETCH**

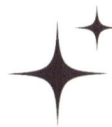

- **HAMSTRINGS & HIP FLEXORS: SIDE SPLITS–** From the Side Split Lunge position, place your back knee and top of your foot on the ground. Straighten your front leg and slowly shift your front foot forward to extend your leg to your maximum stretch. Keep your hands next to your hips. Hold for 10–30 seconds. Reach your hands and arms forward and place your head on your knee. Hold for 10–20 seconds. Repeat on the other side.

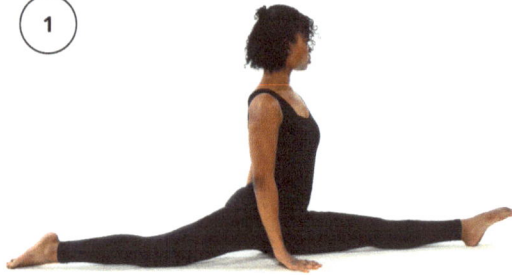

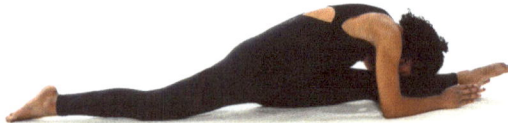

- **HIP FLEXORS: SIDE SPLIT ARCH–** From a Side Split position, place your hands next to your hips, and look back. Start to bend your back from the base of your spine. Focus on getting the crown of your head as close to your back foot as possible. Hold for 10–20 seconds. Repeat on the other side.

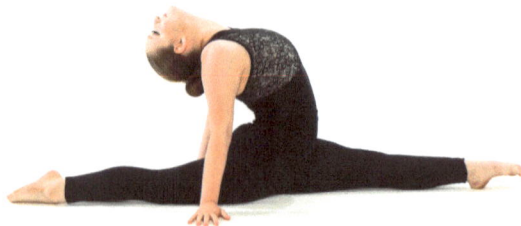

- **HIP FLEXORS: STRADDLE OVER-SPLIT STRETCH-** From a standing position, open your legs into a straddle position and place your hands or forearms down about 1 foot in front of your body with your palms face down on the ground. Open your legs to your maximum Straddle Over-Split Stretch position. With straight legs, rotate externally in your hips with flexed feet and your knees and toes pointing up into the air.

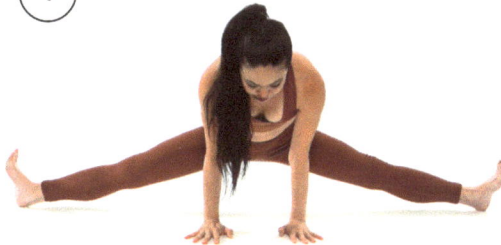

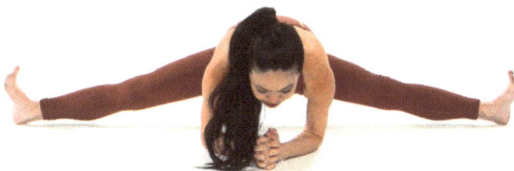

PRO TIP: ENGAGE YOUR QUADRICEPS AND IMAGINE THE MUSCLE LIFTING YOUR KNEE UP TO HELP STRAIGHTEN YOUR LEG

- **GLUTEUS MAXIMUS: BUTTERFLY-** Sit on your sit bones and place the bottoms of your feet together with your knees and hips relaxed to the side. Use your arms or hands to push your knees down to feel the opening in your hips. Forward bend and place your head on your feet. Hold for 10-20 seconds.

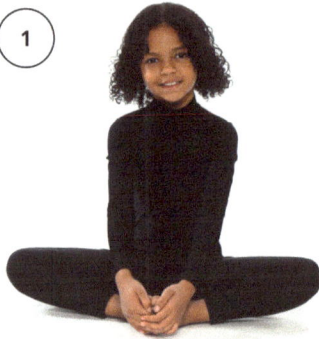
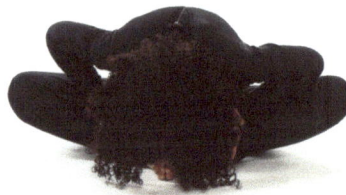

- **GLUTEUS MAXIMUS: BUTTERFLY CROSS-** Once in the Butterfly position, place the top of your right foot on the opposite (or left) knee. Use your right arm to try to push your right knee down to your left foot. Hold for 10-20 seconds and then do it to the other side. For a deeper stretch, forward bend in the Butterfly Cross position.

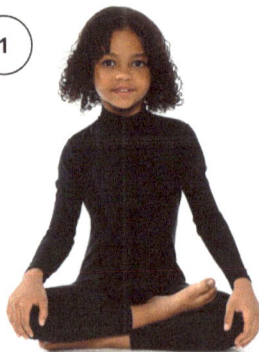
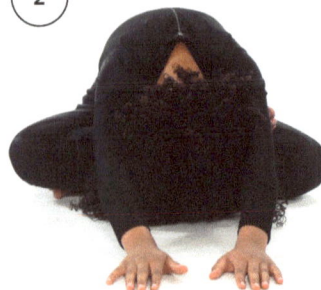

- **GLUTEUS MAXIMUS: BUTTERFLY KNEE CROSS-** Once in the Butterfly Cross position, place the top of your right knee over and across the top of your left knee. Center your knees with the centerline of your body. Hold for 10-20 seconds, then repeat on the other side. Forward bend in the Butterfly Cross position for a deeper stretch.

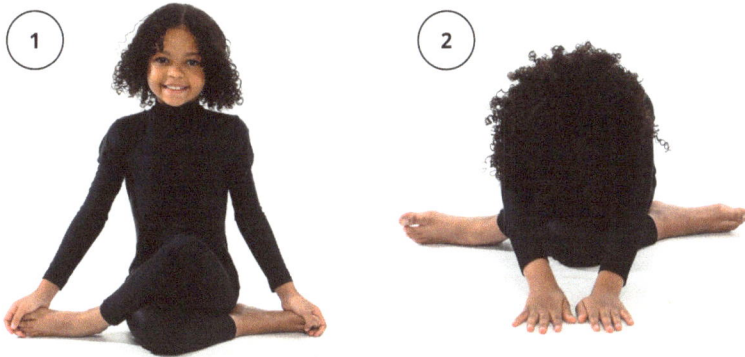

- **BACK & SHOULDER: FLAT BACK-** Stand a little more than hip-width apart. Keep your legs straight, your shoulders down and back, and raise your arms up so they are parallel to the ground next to your ears. From this position fold from your hips to form a flat back. Imagine making a tabletop. Engage your core and legs and hold for 10-20 seconds.

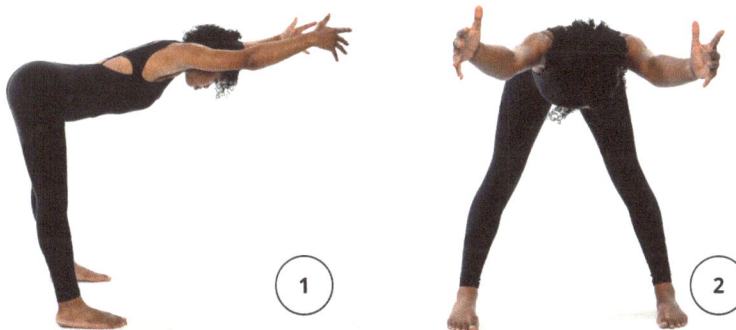

- **BACK: BACKBEND/BRIDGE-** To accomplish a bridge pose, lay down on your back with your knees bent at a 45° angle and your feet placed on the ground hip-width apart. Place your hands beside your ears and point your fingers in the same direction as your toes with your elbows bent. Slowly straighten your arms and legs together as much as possible and hold for 10-20 seconds. Repeat 3-5 times.

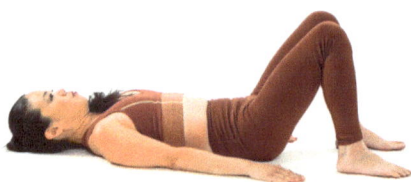
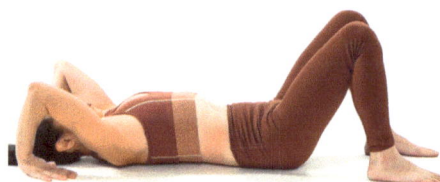

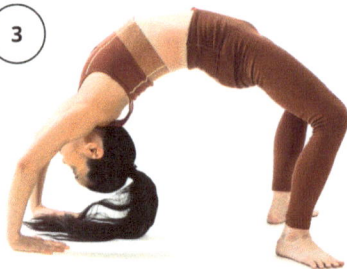
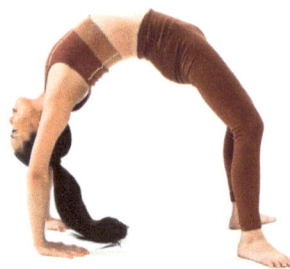

- **BACK: STRAIGHT LEG BRIDGE-** From a Backbend/Bridge position, plant your feet on the ground and straighten your legs. Push your chest over your shoulders and hold for 10-20 seconds.

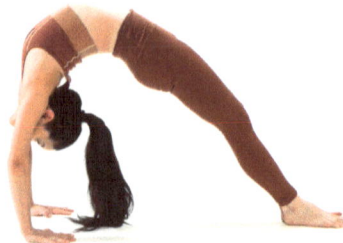

- **BACK: BRIDGE ROCK–** From a Backbend/Bridge position, plant your feet on the ground and push your legs straight to move your chest over your shoulders. Then, bend your legs to shift your weight back toward your legs. Repeat 10 times.

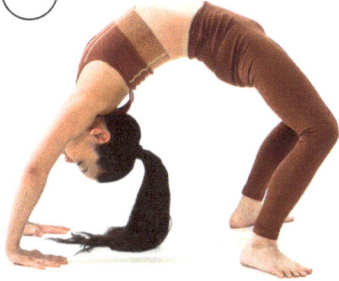 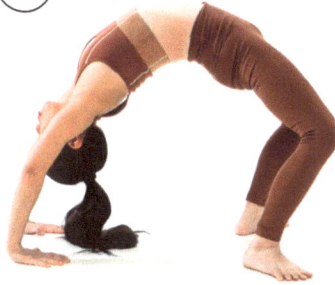

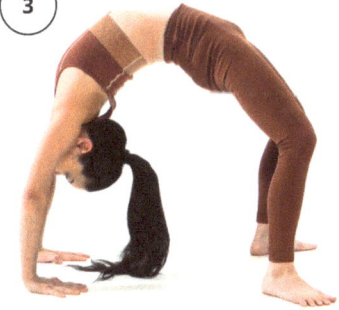 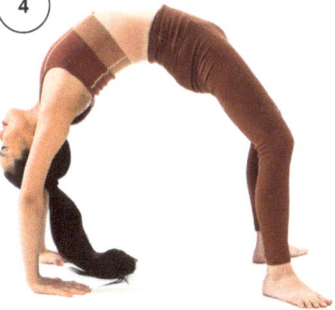

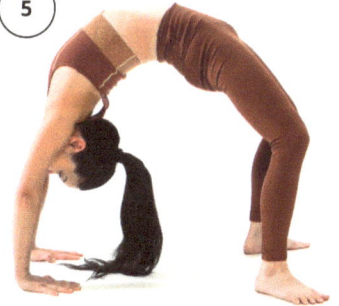 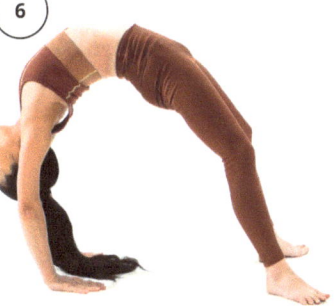

- **BACK & LEGS: BRIDGE SPLIT-** From a Backbend/Bridge position, plant your feet on the ground and bring your right leg and foot to the centerline of the Backbend/Bridge position. Pull your left knee into your chest. When your knee hits the highest point, extend your leg straight. Hold for 10-20 seconds.

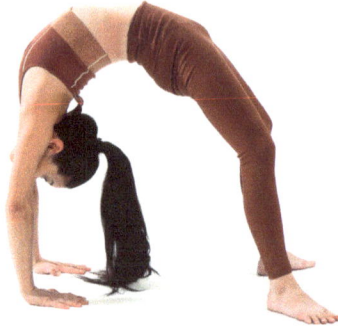

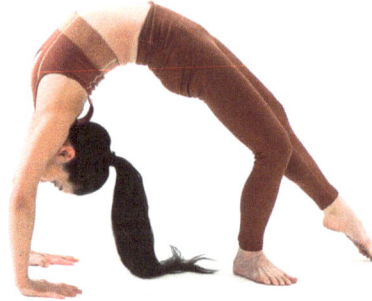

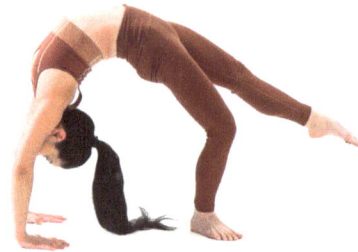

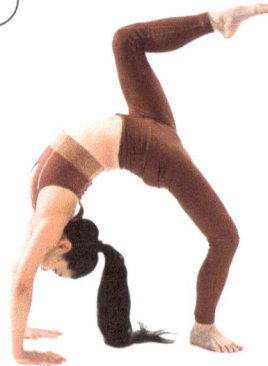

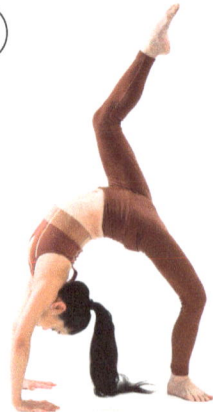

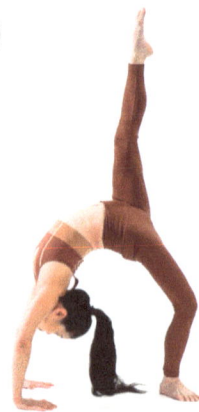

- **BACK & SHOULDER: FOREARM BRIDGE–** From a Backbend/Bridge position, walk your hands forward one at a time to put your forearms down on the ground. Keep your arms parallel and point your fingers toward your feet. Hold for 10–20 seconds. Push back up into a Backbend/Bridge position.

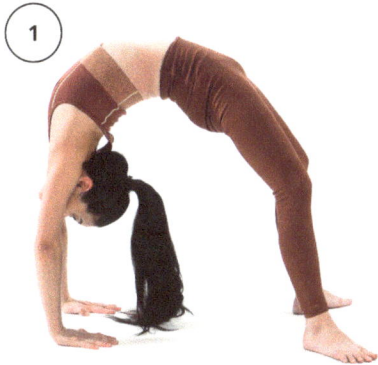

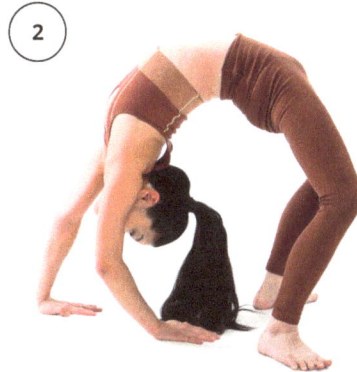

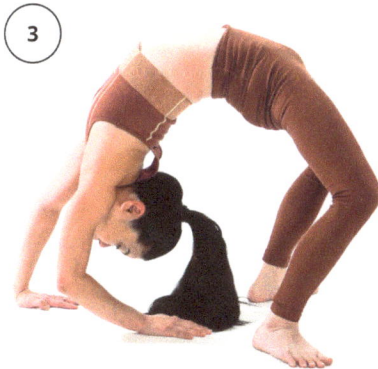

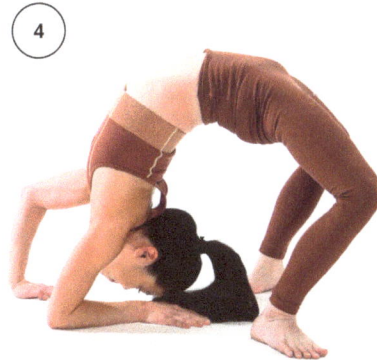

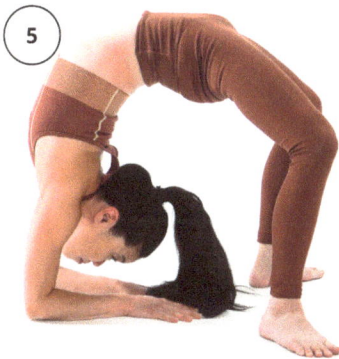

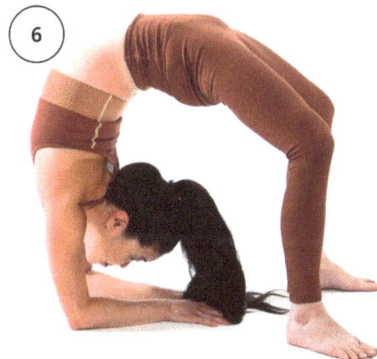

- **LOWER BACK: SEAL POSE-** Lie down on your stomach with your feet at least hip-width apart. Place your hands in a push-up position in alignment with your shoulders. With your hands on the ground, extend your arms straight, keep your shoulders down and back, and look backward. Hold for 10-20 seconds. Repeat 3 times, and bring the legs a little closer together during each round.

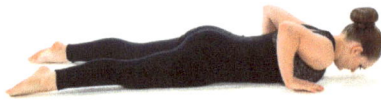

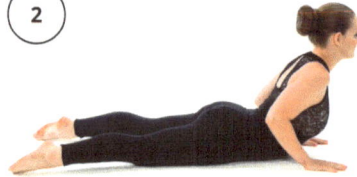

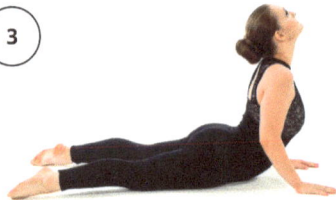

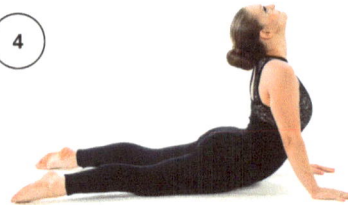

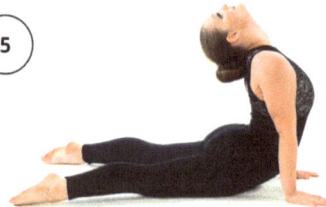

✦

PRO TIP: KEEP WALKING YOUR HANDS CLOSER TO YOUR BODY TO GET A DEEPER STRETCH

✦

- **LOWER BACK: SEAL POSE VARIATION TOES TO HEAD-** Lie down on your stomach with your feet at least hip-width apart. Place your hands in a push-up position in alignment with your shoulders. With your hands on the ground, extend your arms straight, keep your shoulders down and back, and look backward. Bend your knees to bring your toes to your head. Hold for 10-20 seconds. Repeat 3 times, and bring your legs closer together during each round.

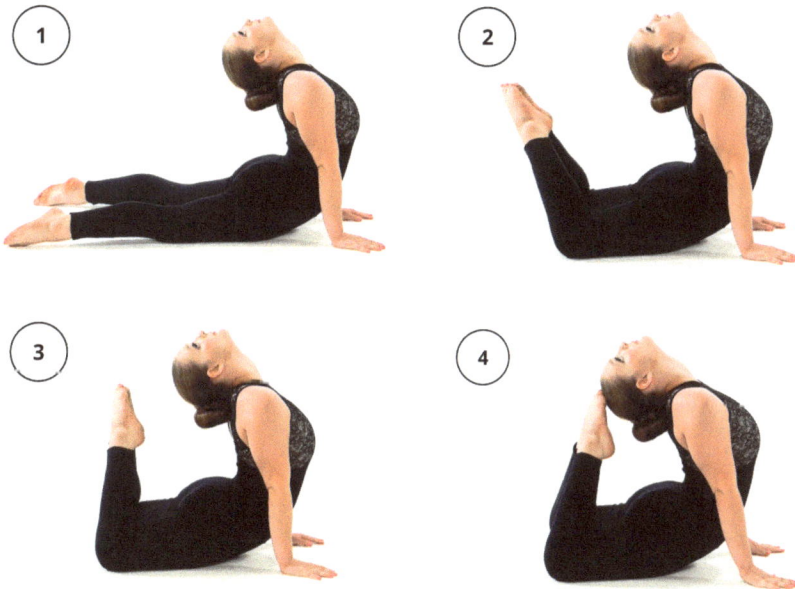

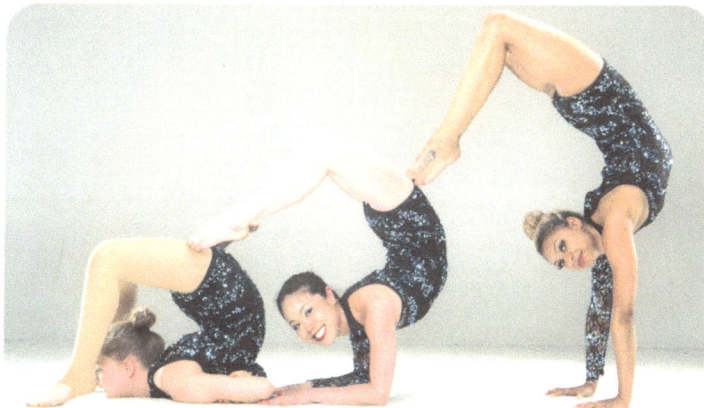

- **LOWER BACK & SHOULDERS: CAMEL POSE–** To begin, move into a kneeling position with your hips and knees in alignment. Slowly lean back and carefully place one hand at a time on the back of your heels with your thumbs toward your pinky toes. Shift your pelvis up and forward and look backward. Remember to relax your neck. Hold for 10–20 seconds. Repeat 2–3 times.

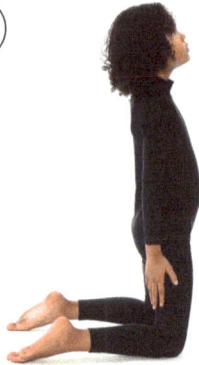
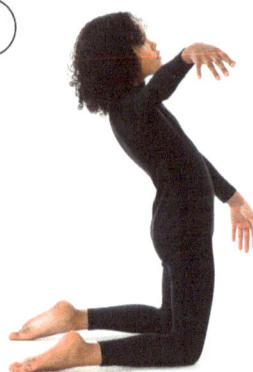

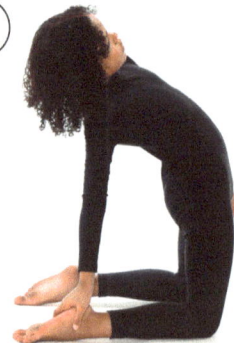
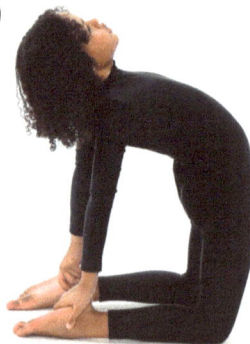

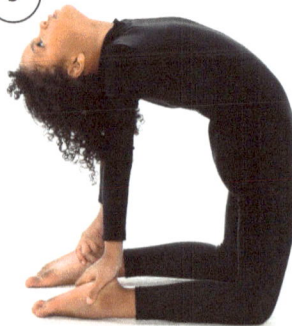

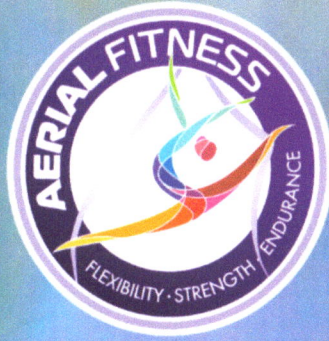

Let's talk splits

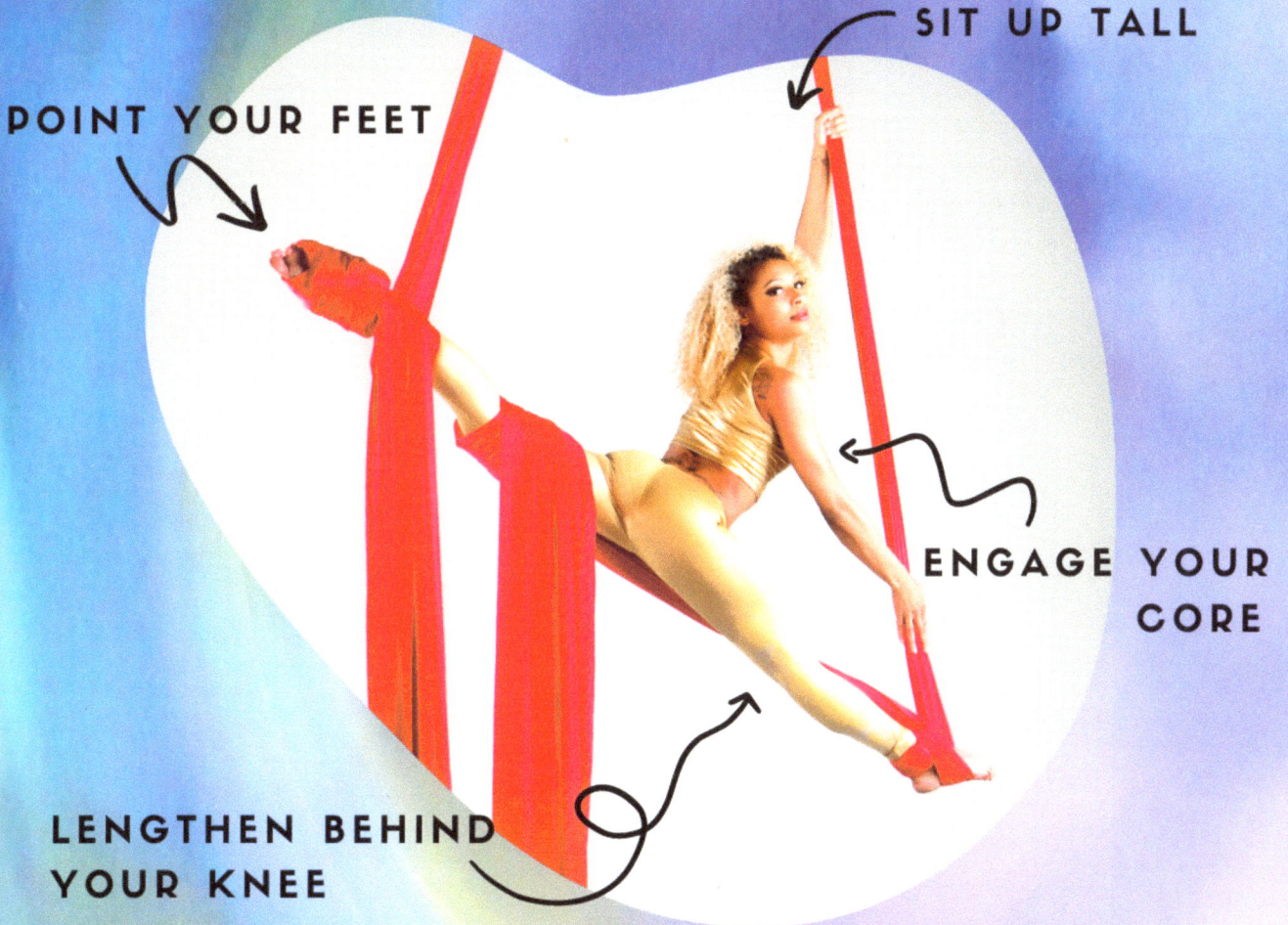

SIT UP TALL

POINT YOUR FEET

ENGAGE YOUR CORE

LENGTHEN BEHIND YOUR KNEE

Cool-Down Routine

Your cool-down routine after your workout is very similar to your warm-up routine, but just at a reduced intensity and a slower pace. Use this time to reflect on what skills you have worked on in your session. Think about the things you can improve on to have better practice in your next session.

Your cool-down routine will also help you break down the lactic acid formation in your body before it has a chance to start to increase. It will also reduce inflammation, which will help with injury prevention.

Repeat the exercises that make your body feel good. Inhale and imagine your breath going into the tightness and pain in your body. Exhale, and release all of the tension that exists.

Your cool-down routine will help your body for the next day's adventures.

LOVE YOURSELF!

LOVE YOUR BODY!

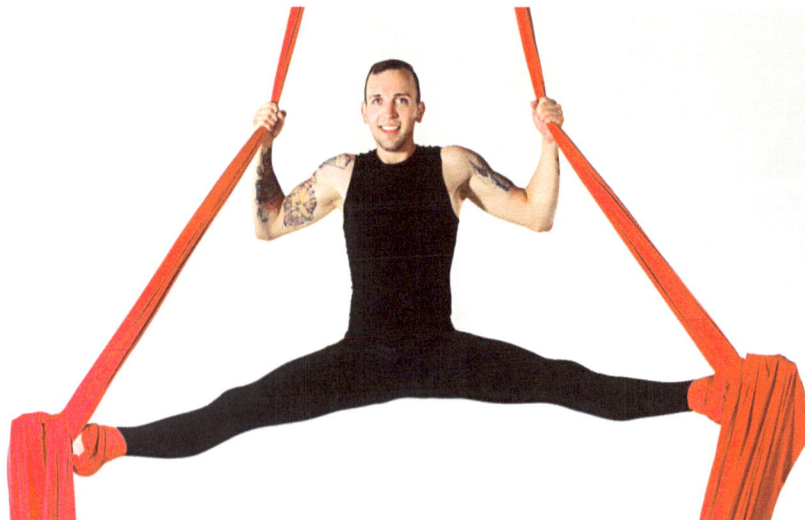

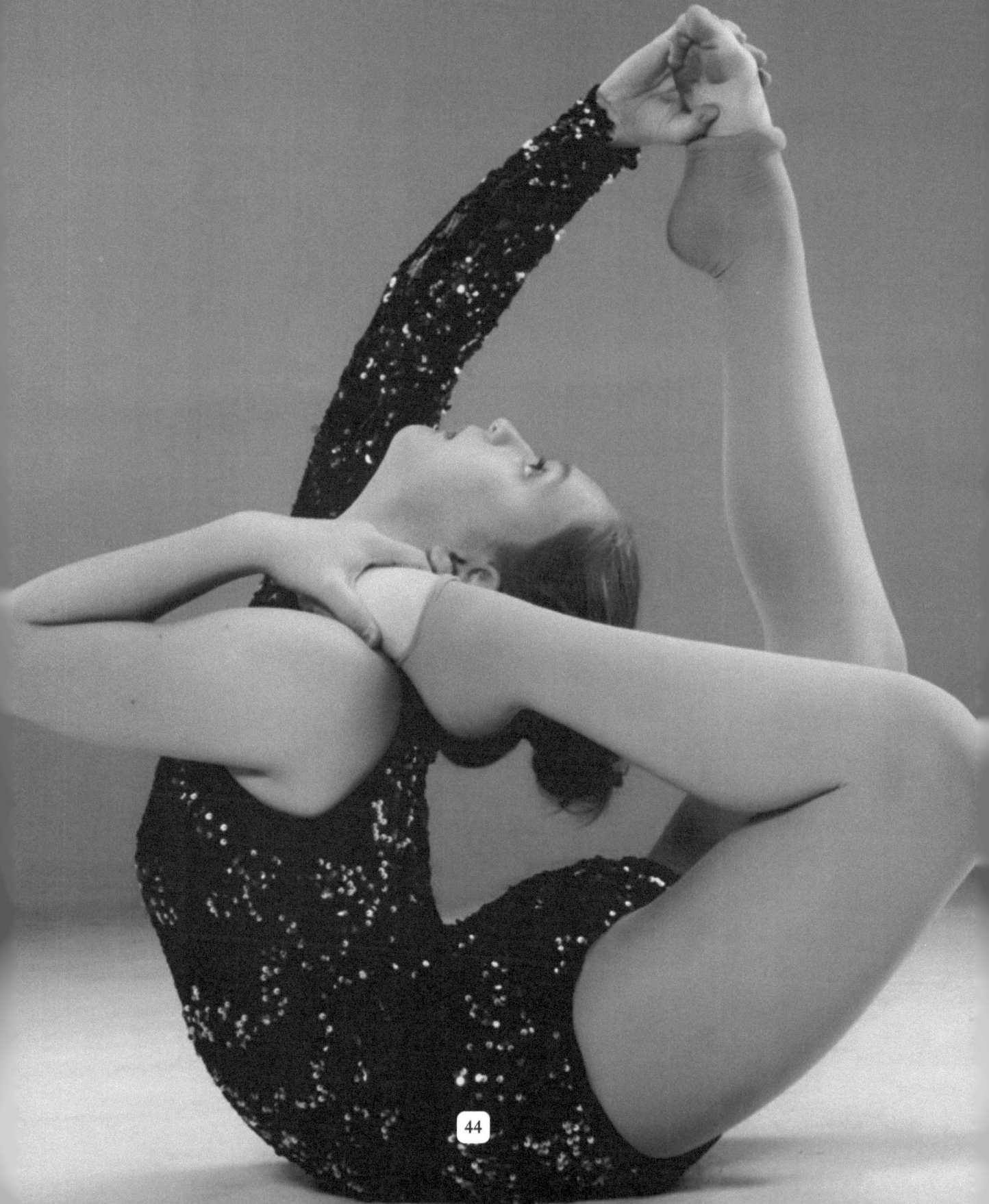

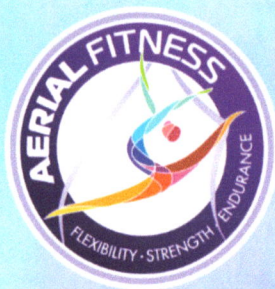

TO DO LIST

to:students	date:today

note:

Train

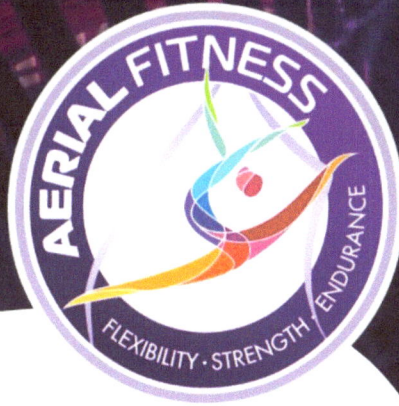

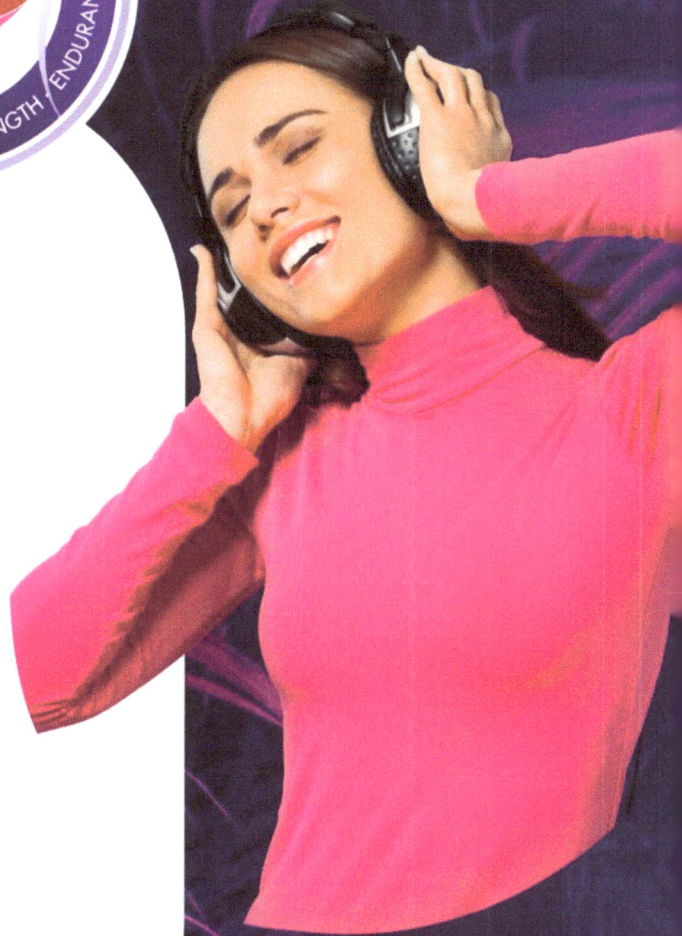

WHY LISTENING TO MUSIC DURING EXERCISE MATTERS

Do you feel powerless while exercising? Try listening to music with your headphones to boost your performance!

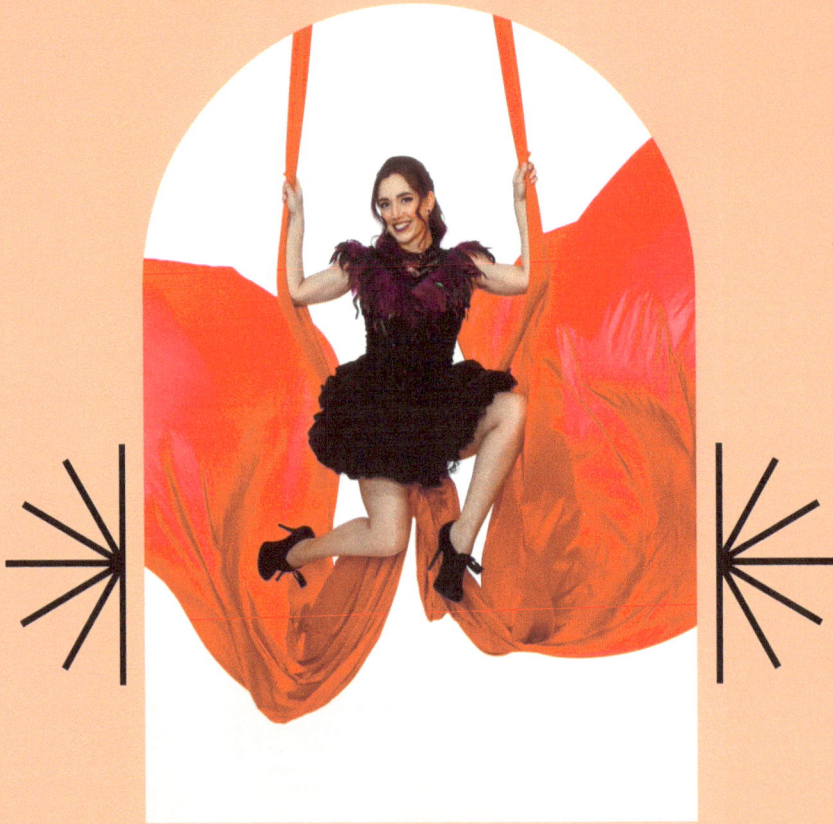

AERIAL FITNESS

AERIAL FITNESS CONDITIONING ROUTINE

Aerial Fitness Conditioning Routine

- **Plank:** Begin in a crawling position, extend your legs back, and place the bottom of your toes on the ground. With a straight spine, glue your feet and legs together. Place your shoulders over your wrists and pull your navel into your spine to engage your core. Your body should be flat and almost parallel to the ground. Hold for 30–60 seconds. Remember to breathe steadily.

- **Push-Ups:** Begin in a Plank position with your hands directly under your shoulders or in a wider stance if desired. Slowly bend the elbows into the body until you are completely parallel to the ground or at your maximum range. Once you are at the lowest point in your position, straighten your arms to push back up. To maintain proper technique, do not drop your belly or sink into your lower back. If this is too difficult, you may place your knees on the ground until you are ready to progress onto your feet. In the beginning, you may have a goal of 5 Push-Ups. Slowly increase in 5 or 10-rep increments until you reach your desired goal. Repeat this exercise with your elbows bent away from the body.

- **Adductor Lifts:** To begin, lie down on your side and pull your navel into your centerline to engage your core. You may rest your head down on your arm or hold your head with your hand. Place your top foot on the ground in front of your pelvis. Flex the foot of your bottom leg and lift your bottom leg toward the sky. Do 1 set of 10, then repeat with a pointed foot. Do 1 set of 10, then repeat on the other side.

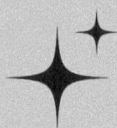

- **Abductor Lifts:** To begin, lie down on your side and pull your navel into your centerline to engage your core. You may rest your head down on your arm or hold your head with your hand. With a straight leg and flexed foot, lift your top leg at least 12 inches and then lower it back down to meet the bottom leg. Do 1 set of 10. Repeat the exercise with a pointed foot, then repeat on the other side.

- **Leg Lifts on back:** To begin, lie down and glue your feet and legs together. Pull your navel into the centerline and press your lower back onto the ground to engage your core. Place your arms by your side with your palms face down. With control, lift your legs. As they approach 90°, lift your hips and touch your toes on the ground above your head. After you reach your maximum, slowly lower your spine one vertebra at a time as you lower your legs back to the ground. Do 1 set of 10. Keep your legs straight the whole time. For more of a challenge, interlace your fingers and raise your arms over your head.

- **Oblique Leg Lifts on Back:** To begin, lie down and glue your feet and legs together. Pull your navel into the centerline and press your lower back onto the ground to engage your core. Place your arms to the side perpendicular to your body so it makes a "T". Pull your knees up into your chest until your legs are at a 90° angle. Glue your legs together and lower them to the right side until your legs touch the ground. Then lift your legs to the left side to complete one set. Do 1 set of 10. For more of a challenge, do this exercise with straight legs.

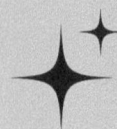

- **Back Extensions:** To begin, lie on your stomach and glue your feet and legs together. Pull your navel into your spine to engage your core. Place your hands behind your head and interlock your fingers and point your elbows out toward the sides of your body. Lift your upper body as high as possible with your pelvis and legs glued to the ground. When you reach your highest point, lower your upper body back to the ground with control. Do 1 set of 10.

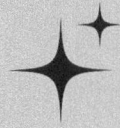

Aerial Fitness Core Relationship

In any Aerial Fitness movement, you must always be conscious of activating your core muscle groups. This will help you strengthen your body in your workout and make you feel and appear 'lighter' in the air. When you activate your core muscles, it will be easier to move, you will have more stability in the air, and the aerial silk or rigging will also not swing, twist, or vibrate as much or at all. As your core strengthens, you will gain more control over the aerial silk. Always remember to activate your core muscles during the Aerial Fitness workout.

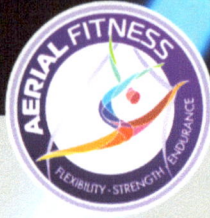

DID YOU KNOW?

- ✓ Exercising improves brain performance.

- ✓ Working out sharpens your memory.

- ✓ Exercise prevents signs of aging

- ✓ Exercising boosts self-confidence

- ✓ Working out enables you to sleep better

KRISTI TOGUCHI

AERIAL FITNESS® TECHNIQUE

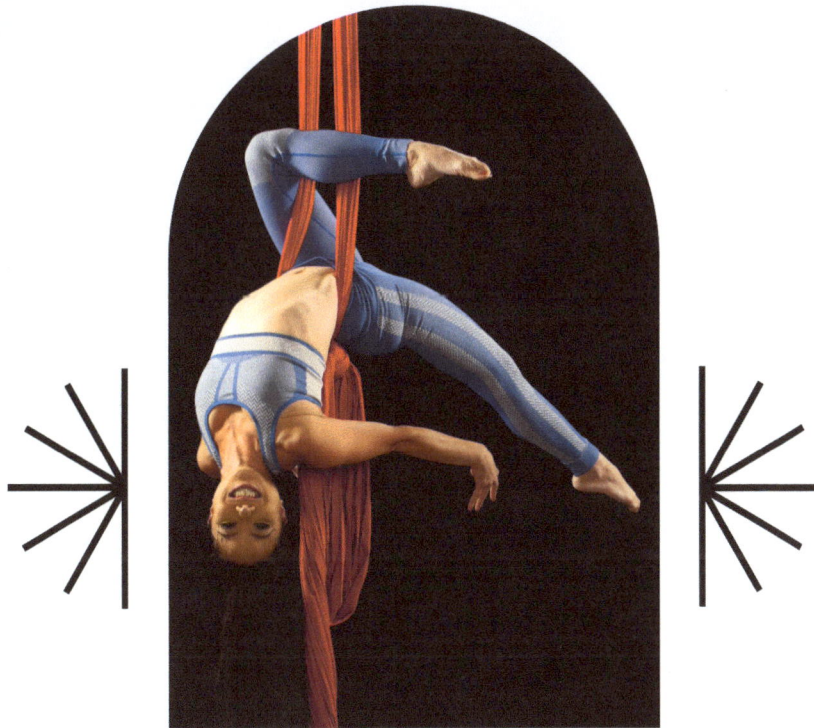

AERIAL FITNESS

FUNDAMENTALS

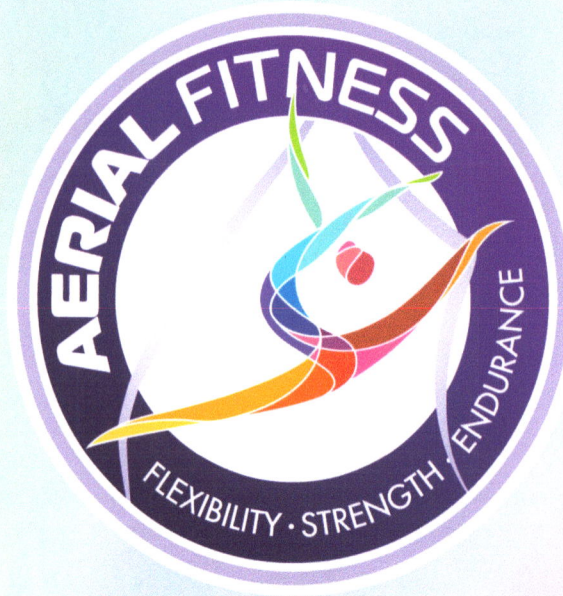

Aerial Fitness
warm-up, cool-down, and conditioning
exercises for all fitness levels.

PROCEED AT YOUR OWN RISK

AERIAL FITNESS

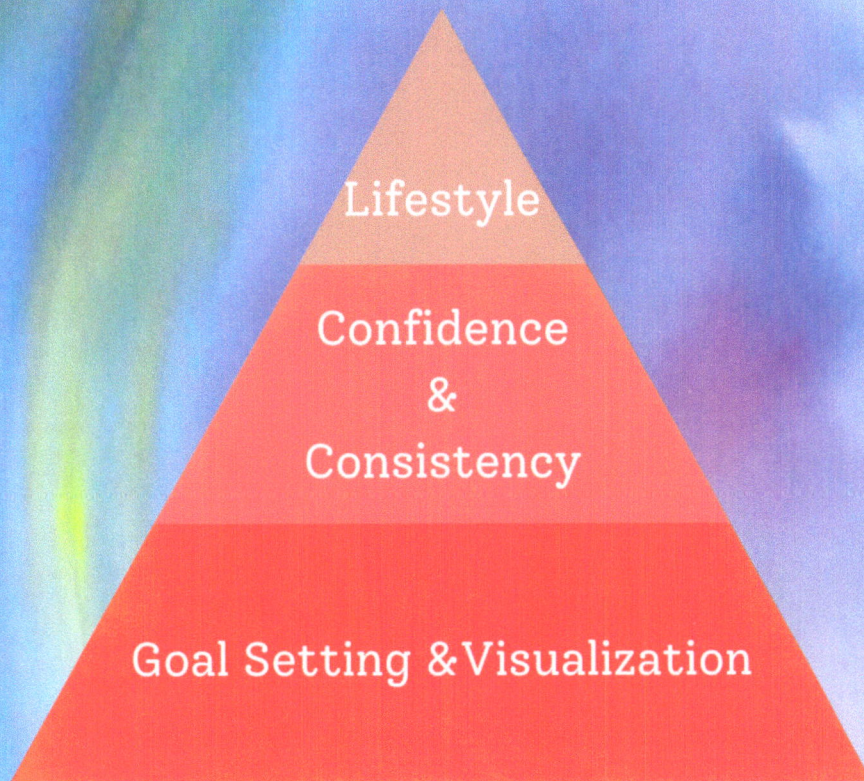

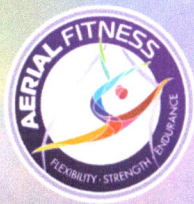

Lifestyle

Confidence
&
Consistency

Goal Setting & Visualization

AERIAL FITNESS

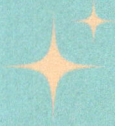

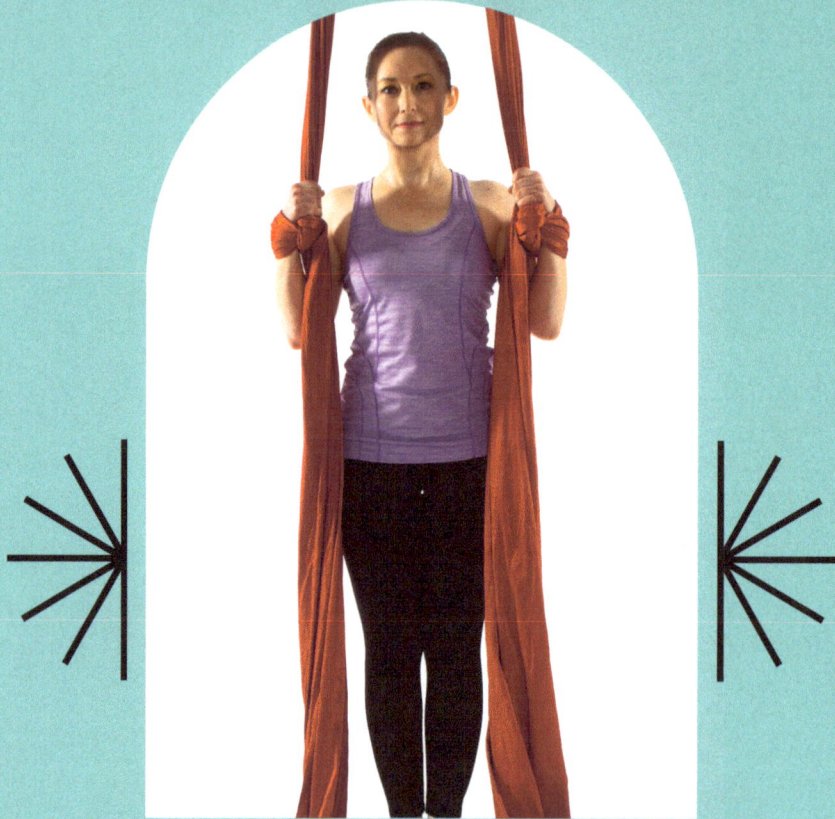

HAND KNOT TECHNIQUE

Learning to tie knots with the aerial silk fabric will increase the level of safety as you are learning the foundations of the Aerial Fitness workout.

55

The Aerial Silk Hand Knot provides additional support to build the tiny muscles in the hands you need to grip the fabric. First, split the fabric and hug each fabric with your hands up into the air. With the right hand, pick up the fabric that dangles under the left hand. Bring the fabric over your wrist from your thumb to your pinky finger. The fabric will create an "X" over the top of your wrist. Then grip the fabric above the Aerial Silk Hand Knot and repeat with the other hand. It is important to remember that although the knots provide additional support, they are not a harness. You must still hold onto the fabric for safety to ensure you do not fall. As you get stronger, you can eliminate the knots and use wraps or pure grip strength.

AERIAL SILK HAND KNOT

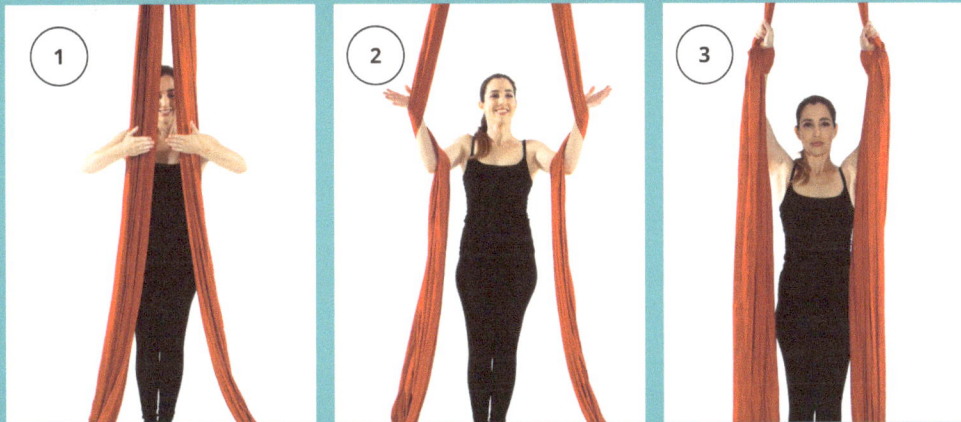

Aerial Silk Hand Wrap: To begin, stand and face the fabric. Split the fabric and start to hug each fabric with your hands up in the air.

Wrap your wrists again to create a double wrap on each wrist. Then grip the fabric with your hands above the two wraps around your wrists.

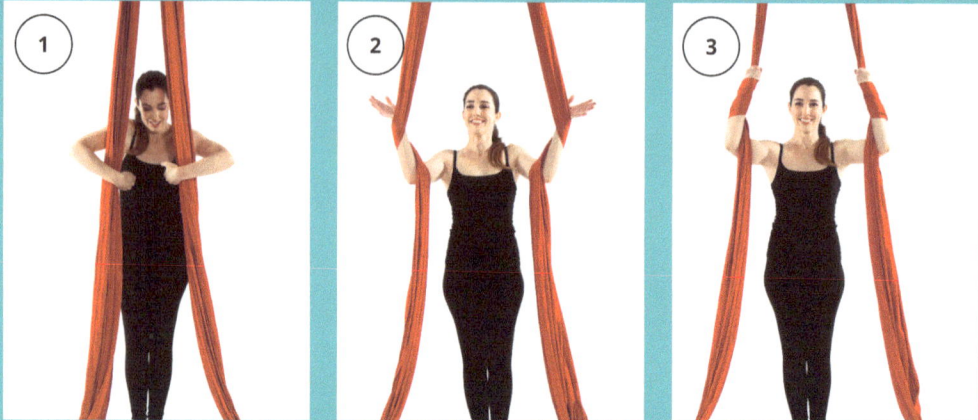

As you build strength in your hands, the next progression is a handgrip. To begin, stand and face the fabric. Split the fabric with your fingers together and create a hook with your hands. Pull your shoulders down and back. Align your wrists with your arms, so you do not collapse or twerk at the wrists. Grip the fabric with hooked hands and close it off with your thumbs.

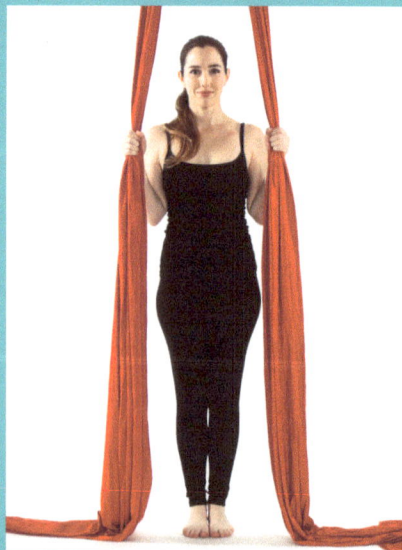

HAND KNOT PLANK

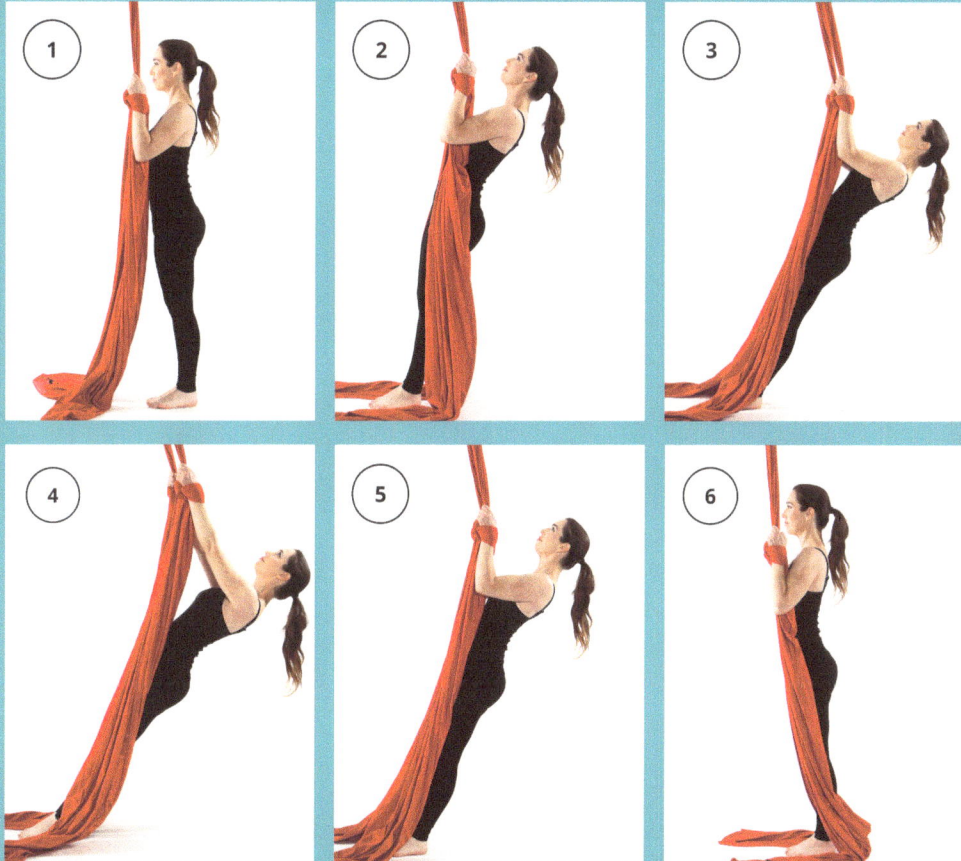

To begin, tie hand knots evenly about shoulder height. Glue your legs together, feet together, and pull your navel into your spine. Make sure to pull your shoulders down and back. Use your core muscles to keep your body in a straight position the whole time. Try not to bend in your knees or lower back. Hold onto the aerial silk and slowly lean back and lower your body with control until your arms are fully extended. Once your body is in your deepest plank position, pull yourself back up to the original standing position. Do 1 set of 10.

HAND KNOT SHOULDER SHRUG

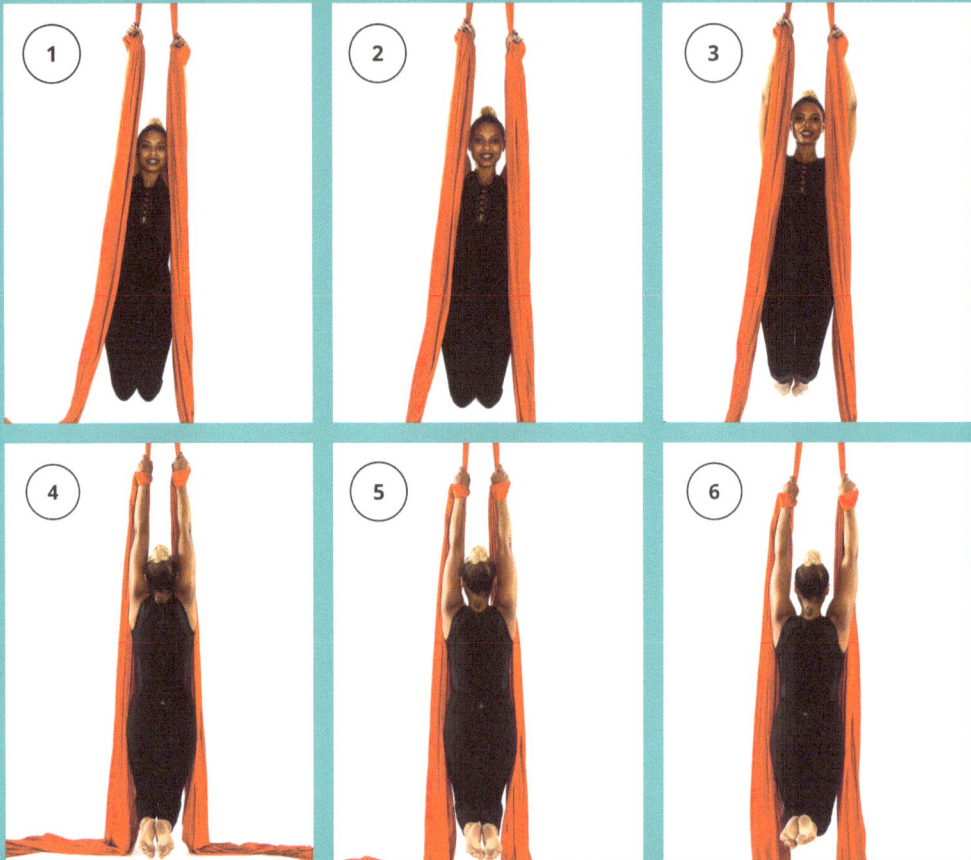

To begin, tie hand knots evenly as high as you comfortably can. Glue your legs together, feet together, and pull your navel into your spine. Make sure to use your latissimus dorsi muscle (largest back muscle) to pull your shoulders down and back. It is essential to engage your back muscles the entire time. Try not to let your shoulders rise toward your ears. Bend at your knees to lift your legs off the ground so your body is in a hanging position. Once in a hanging position, begin to use your latissimus dorsi muscle to shrug your shoulders up toward your ears and then down and back. Do 2–5 sets of 10. For more of a challenge, you can hold your legs in the pike position.

HAND KNOT TUCK

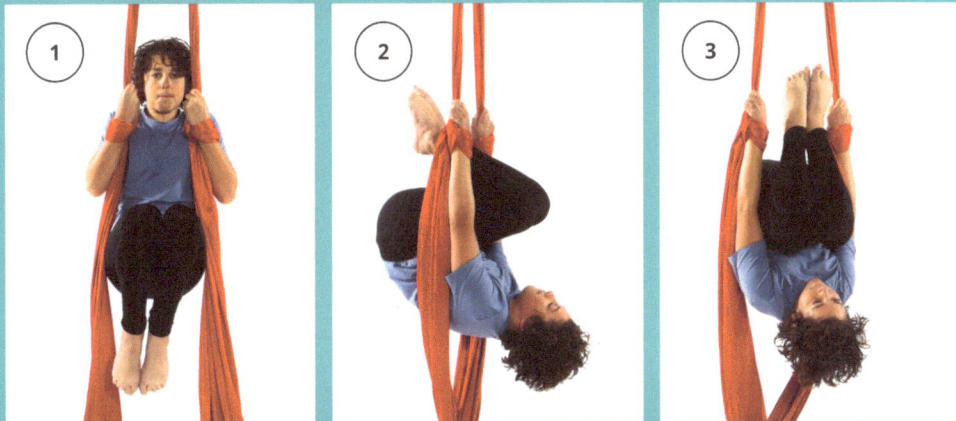

To begin, tie hand knots evenly about shoulder height. Glue your legs together, feet together, and pull your navel into your spine. Make sure to use your latissimus dorsi muscle (largest back muscle) to pull your shoulders down and back. Imagine doing a chin-up on a bar between your two hands. Then pick up your legs into a tuck position pulling your knees into your chest. Start to lean back and extend the arms to move your legs and pelvis above your head. Hold for 10 seconds.

If this is too difficult, start from a seated position and use the fabric above your hand knots as a bar. Try to get up one leg at a time by trapping your foot or leg on the fabric above your hands. Once you are balanced, try to take off one leg at a time and move it into the tuck position and hold for 10 seconds. As you build strength and awareness, you should try to tie your hand knots progressively higher and use your muscles to control the movement.

HAND KNOT HANDSTAND

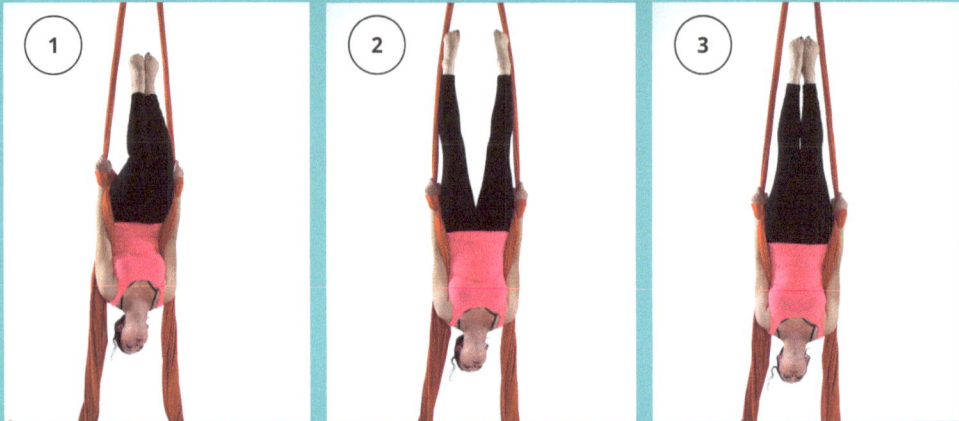

To begin, tie hand knots evenly about shoulder height. Glue your legs together, feet together, and pull your navel into your spine. Make sure to use your latissimus dorsi muscle (largest back muscle) to pull your shoulders down and back. Move into the Hand Knot Tuck position. From the tuck position, raise your legs into the handstand position. Hold for 10 seconds.

If this is too difficult, try to use the fabric as a spot by pushing your feet against it to create tension. This will allow you to raise your legs with the assistance of the aerial silk. Once your legs are fully extended up into the air, try to bring your legs to the center one leg at a time into the full handstand position. Hold for 10 seconds.

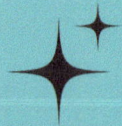

PRO TIP: USE PROGRESSIONS AND MODIFY EXERCISES ACCORDING TO YOUR CURRENT ABILITY

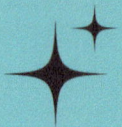

HAND KNOT PIKE

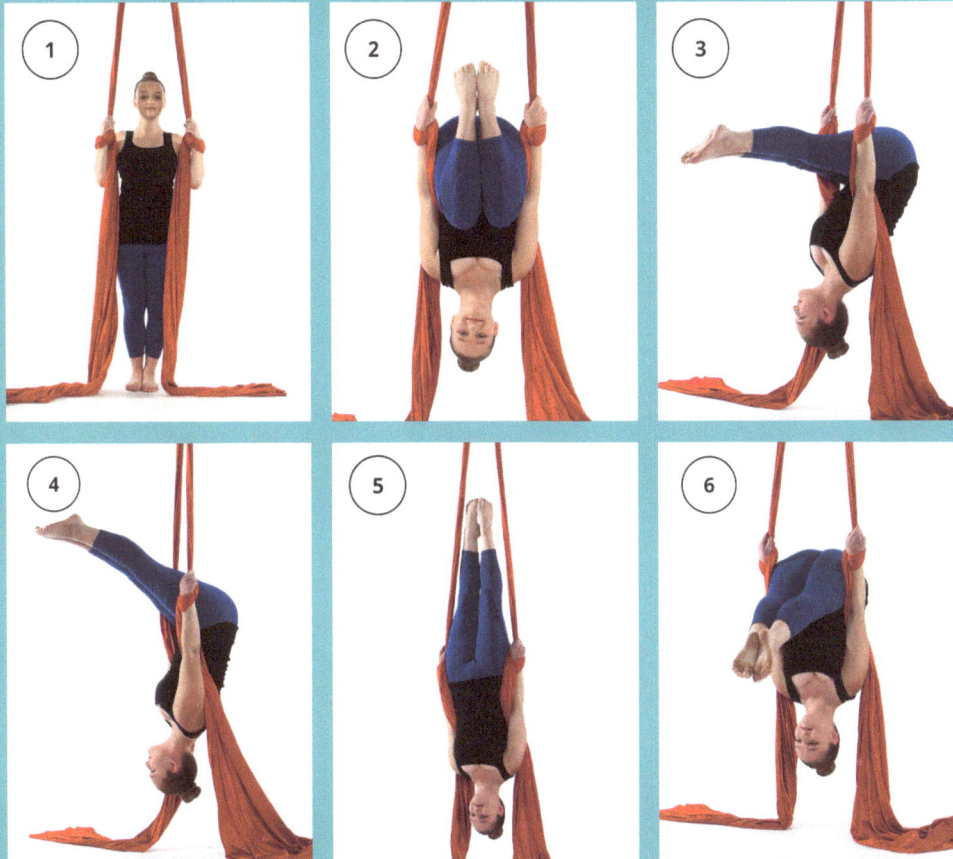

To begin, tie hand knots evenly about shoulder height. Glue your legs together, feet together, and pull your navel into your spine. Make sure to use your latissimus dorsi muscle (largest back muscle) to pull your shoulders down and back. Move into the Hand Knot Tuck position. To pike, extend your legs forward, creating a 90° angle with your body or an "L" shape. Raise your legs into a handstand position. Then lower your legs back into the pike position. Do 1 set of 10.

HAND KNOT RUNS

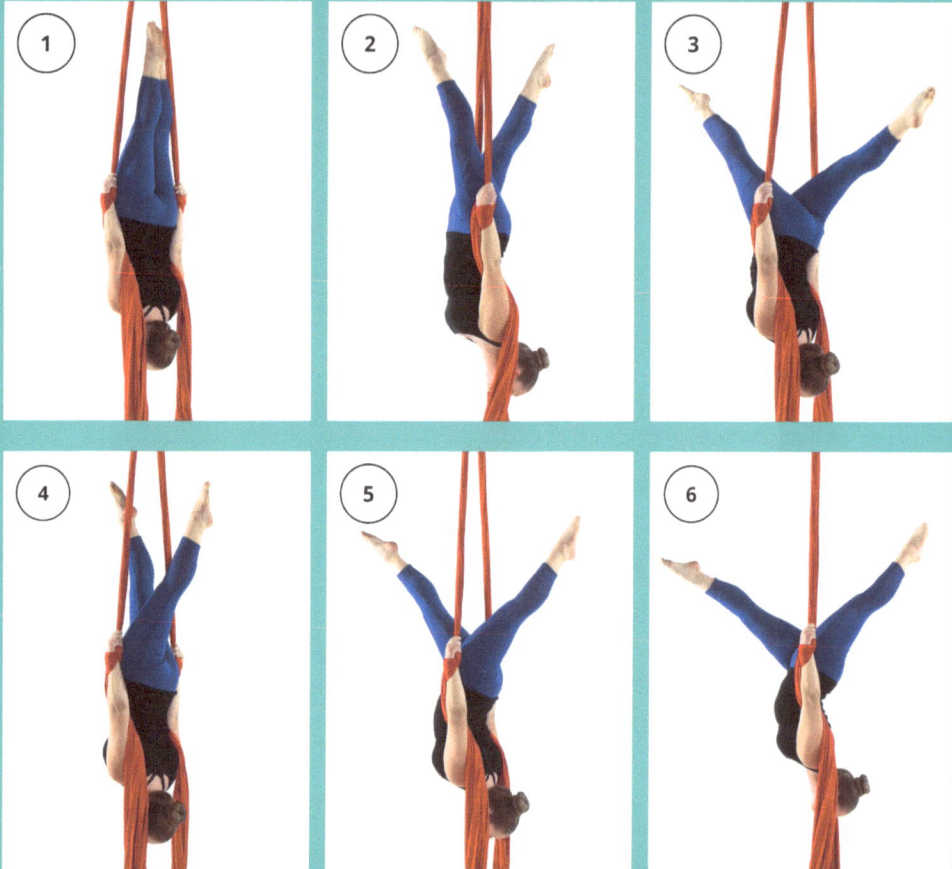

To begin, tie hand knots evenly about shoulder height. Glue your legs together, feet together, and pull your navel into your spine. Make sure to use your latissimus dorsi muscle (largest back muscle) to pull your shoulders down and back. Move into the Hand Knot Handstand position. Start to scissor the legs front and back, with straight legs. Make sure to open your legs evenly and on the centerline. As you gain control, strength, and flexibility, try to open your legs wider and wider. Do 1 set of 10.

HAND KNOT SPLITS

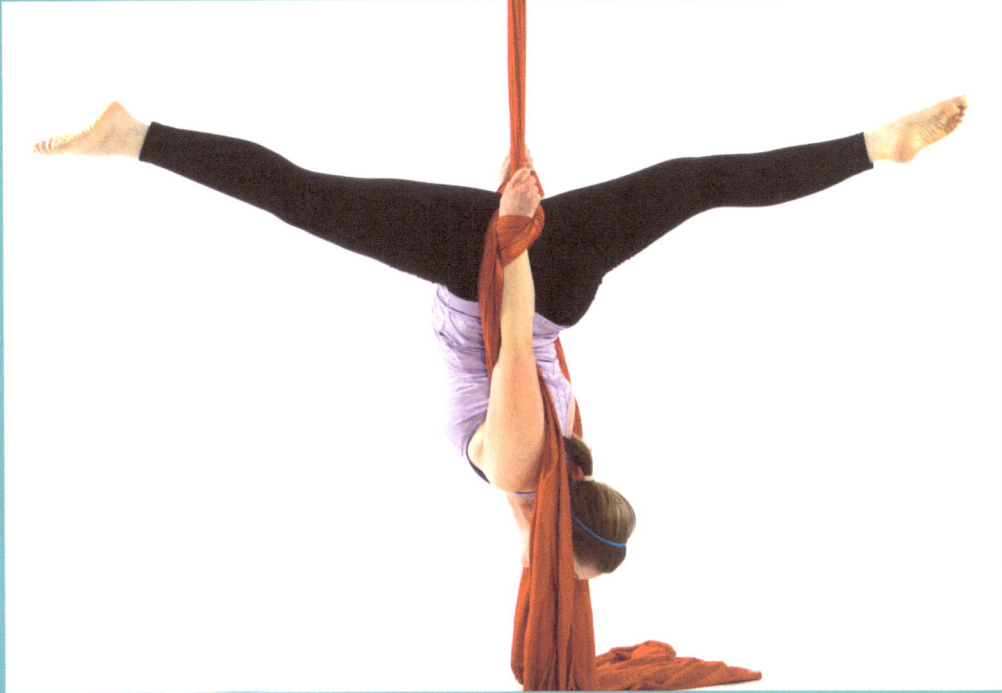

To begin, tie hand knots evenly about shoulder height. Glue your legs together, feet together, and pull your navel into your spine. Make sure to use your latissimus dorsi muscle (largest back muscle) to pull your shoulders down and back. Move into the Hand Knot Handstand position. Start to open your legs like a scissor from front to back. Make sure to spread your legs evenly and on the centerline. Once your legs are extended to their maximum, hold for 10 seconds. Repeat to the other side.

To add a back and neck stretch to your Hand Knot Split, open your legs to their maximum, bend your back, and look backward. Hold for 10 seconds. Repeat to the other side.

HAND KNOT SPLIT STAG

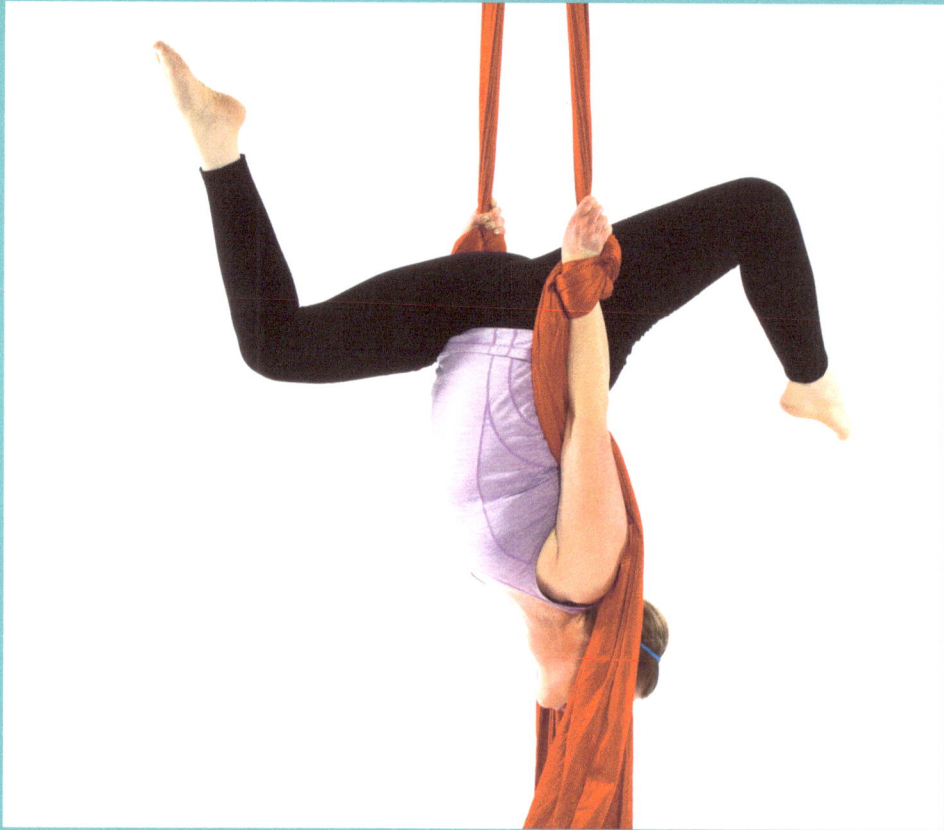

To begin, tie hand knots evenly about shoulder height. Glue your legs together, feet together, and pull your navel into your spine. Make sure to use your latissimus dorsi muscle (largest back muscle) to pull your shoulders down and back. Move into the Hand Knot Split position. Bend both legs at about a 90° angle. Hold for 10 seconds. Repeat to the other side.

To add a back and neck stretch to your Hand Knot Split Stag position, bend your back, and look backward. Hold for 10 seconds. Repeat to the other side.

HAND KNOT BIRD'S NEST

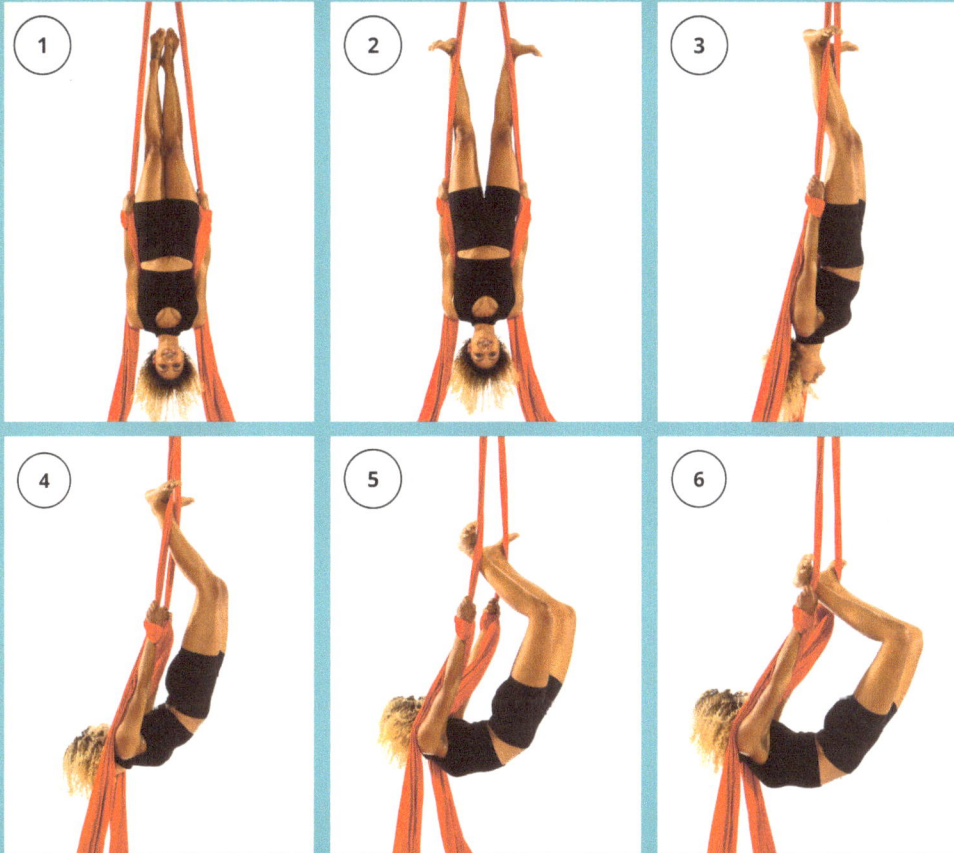

To begin, tie hand knots evenly about shoulder height. Glue your legs together, feet together, and pull your navel into your spine. Make sure to use your latissimus dorsi muscle (largest back muscle) to pull your shoulders down and back. Move into the Hand Knot Handstand position. Flex your feet and place your feet on the backside of the fabric from where you are facing. Start to move your feet to your hands as you bend your back and lift your head. Bend your knees on the inside of the fabric and release your pelvis forward into the ground into a bridge or backbend-like position in the air. When at your maximum stretch, hold for 10 seconds.

HAND KNOT
BIRD'S NEST SPLIT

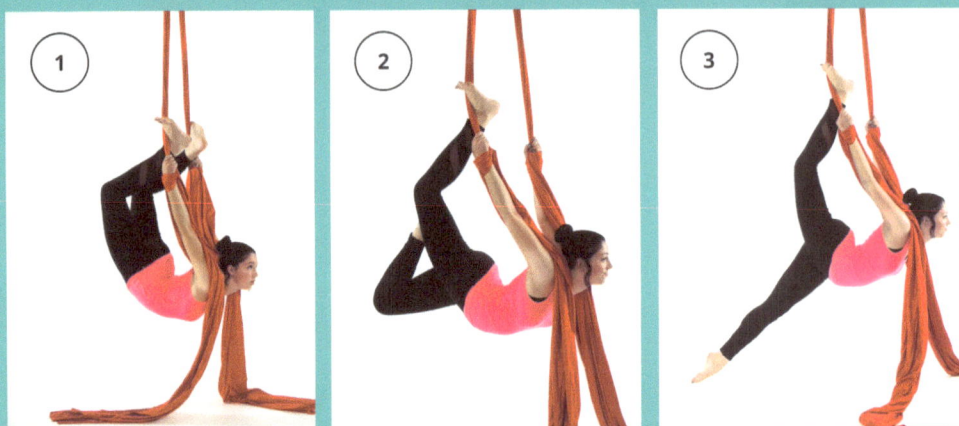

To begin, tie hand knots evenly about shoulder height. Glue your legs together, feet together, and pull your navel into your spine. Make sure to use your latissimus dorsi muscle (largest back muscle) to pull your shoulders down and back. Move into the Hand Knot Bird's Nest position. With control, take one foot off the fabric and lower the foot to the ground into a split position. Keep your head up and have your other leg maintain the original Hand Knot Bird's Nest position. Hold for 10 seconds. Repeat to the other side.

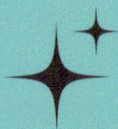

✦

PRO TIP: EXTEND THE TOP LEG UP THE FABRIC WITH A STRAIGHT LEG TO ACHIEVE A FULL SPLIT

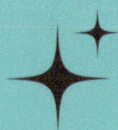

✦

Hand Knot Tuck Crunch Hold

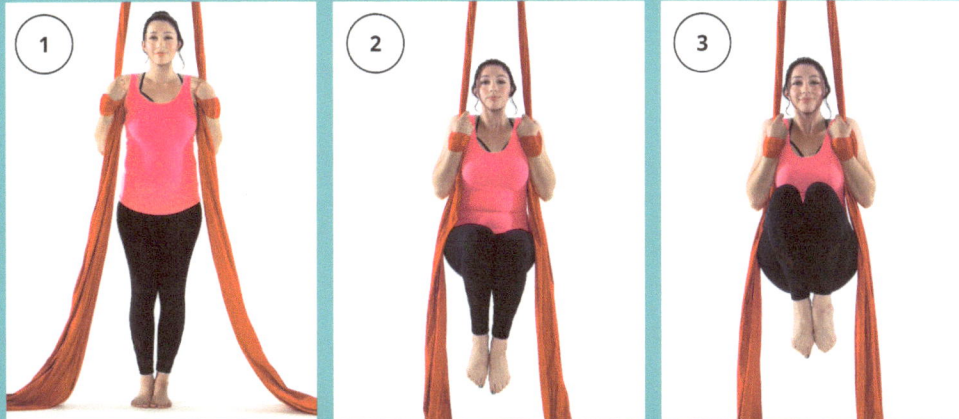

To begin, tie hand knots evenly about shoulder height. Glue your legs together, feet together, and pull your navel into your spine. Make sure to use your latissimus dorsi muscle (largest back muscle) to pull your shoulders down and back. Pull your knees into your chest into a tuck position and hold for 10, 20, 30, or 60 seconds. As you build strength, begin to progressively increase your hold time.

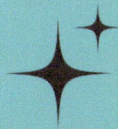

PRO TIP: BUILDING A CORE CONDITIONING ROUTINE ON THE GROUND WILL MAKE MOVEMENTS EASIER WHEN IN THE AIR

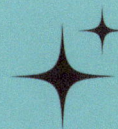

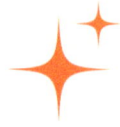

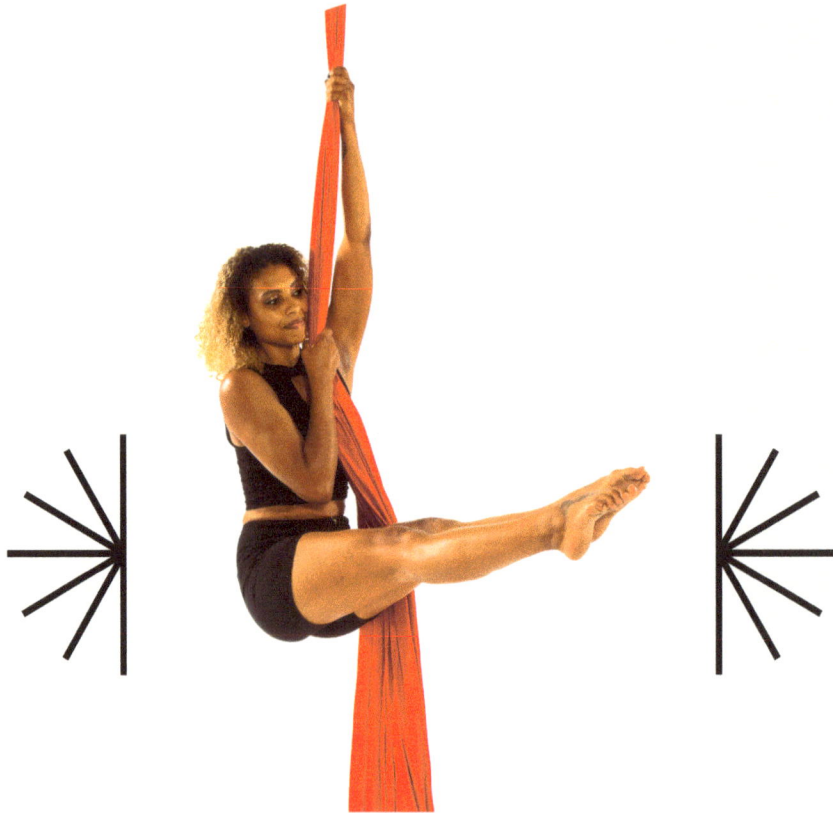

AERIAL FITNESS

CONDITIONING TECHNIQUE

Utilizing progressions of core conditioning will build a strong foundation while developing the muscles necessary to accomplish more challenging exercises.

TUCK CRUNCH

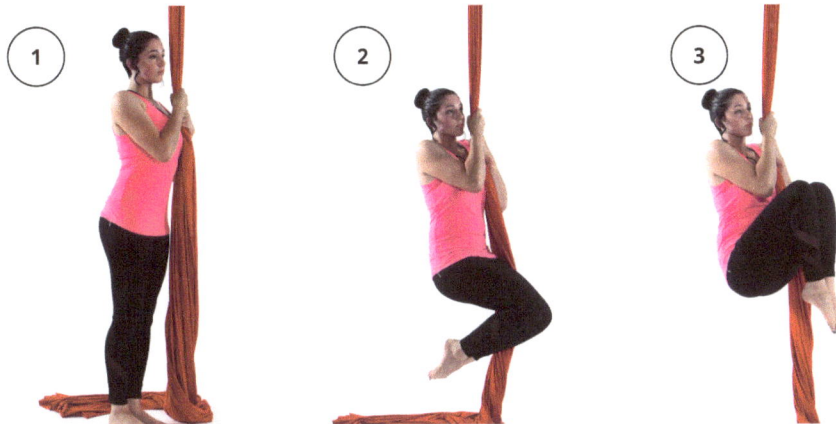

To begin, grab the fabric around or above shoulder height. Glue your legs together, feet together, and pull your navel into your spine. While holding onto the fabric, pull your body up with your hands into your heart. Make sure to use your latissimus dorsi muscle to pull your shoulders down and back. Pull your knees into your chest into a tuck position ten times, trying not to touch the ground again.

If this is too difficult, from the starting position with your hands in front of your heart, jump into a tuck position and touch the ground until you build the strength to do it with proper form.

PROGRESSION: One extended arm handhold.

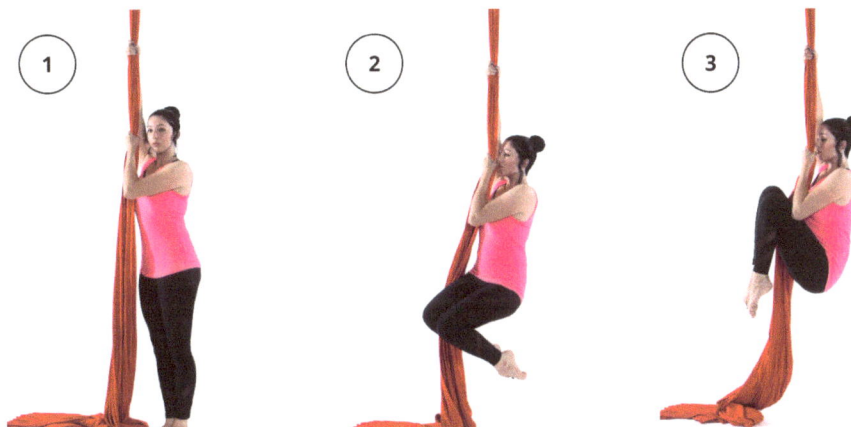

Tuck Crunch Variation

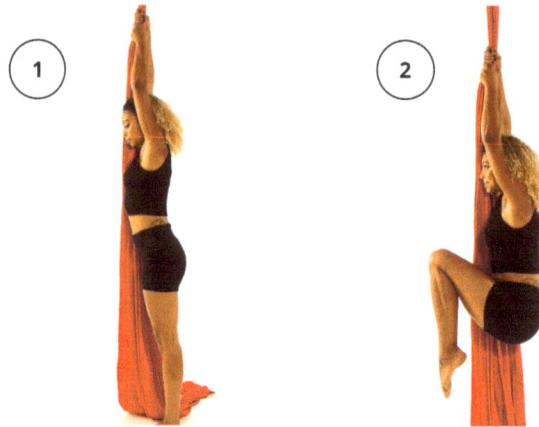

To begin, lift your arms up and grab the fabric above you. Glue your legs together, feet together, and pull your navel into your spine. Make sure to use your latissimus dorsi muscle to pull your shoulders down and back. Hold onto the fabric and pull your knees into your chest into a tuck position ten times, trying not to touch the ground again.

PRO TIP: DON'T FORGET YOUR SELF-CARE PRACTICE BY ACKNOWLEDGING YOUR ACHIEVEMENTS AFTER TRAINING

STRAIGHT LEG LIFTS

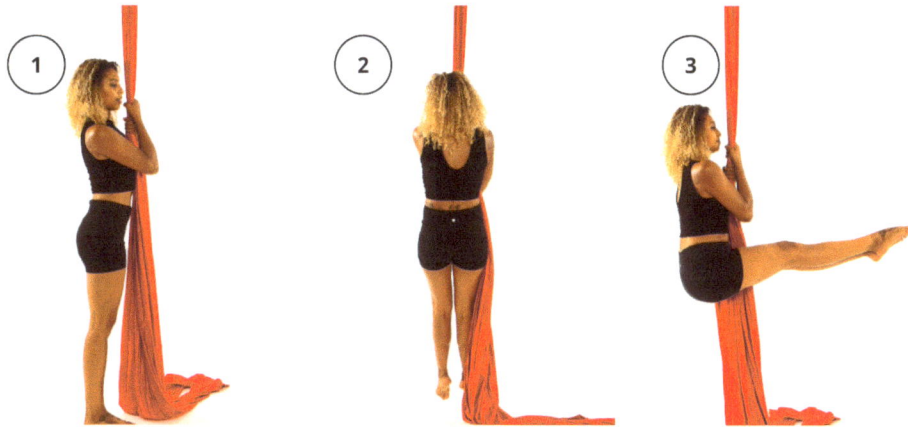

To begin, grab the fabric around or above shoulder height. Glue your legs together, feet together, and pull your navel into your spine. Hold onto the fabric and pull your body up with straight legs and your hands into your heart. Make sure to use your latissimus dorsi muscle to pull your shoulders down and back. With your hands in front of your chest, bring your legs up to a 45° position, then slowly lower your legs to the starting position. Do 1 set of 10.

For more of a challenge, do this exercise by raising your legs to a 90° position. As you build strength, you will be able to progress to the full range of the pike position by raising your legs to a 180° position.

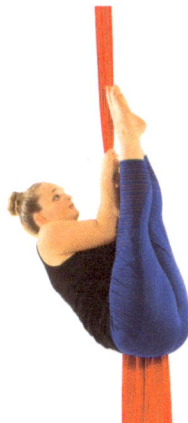

PIKE HOLD

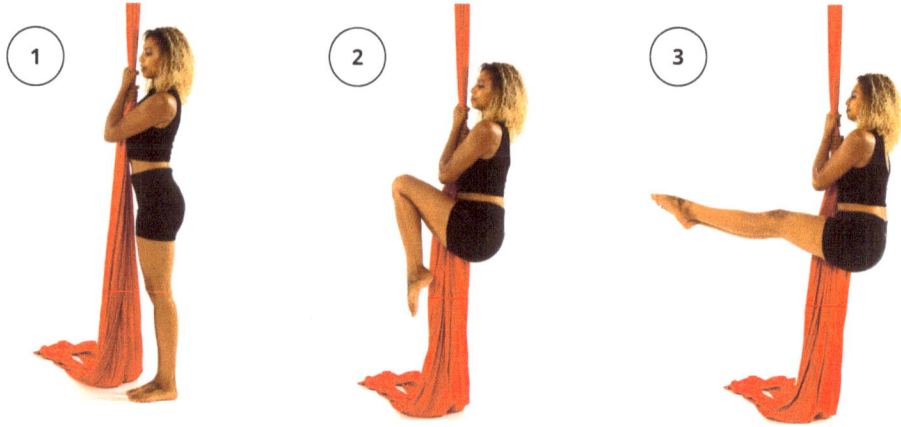

To begin, grab the fabric around or above shoulder height. Glue your legs together, feet together, and pull your navel into your spine. Hold onto the fabric. Make sure to use your latissimus dorsi muscle to pull your shoulders down and back. From a tuck position, extend your legs forward into an "L" sit or a 90° pike position. Hold for 10,20,30, or 60 seconds.

VARIATIONS: Straight arm hang, one extended arm handhold.

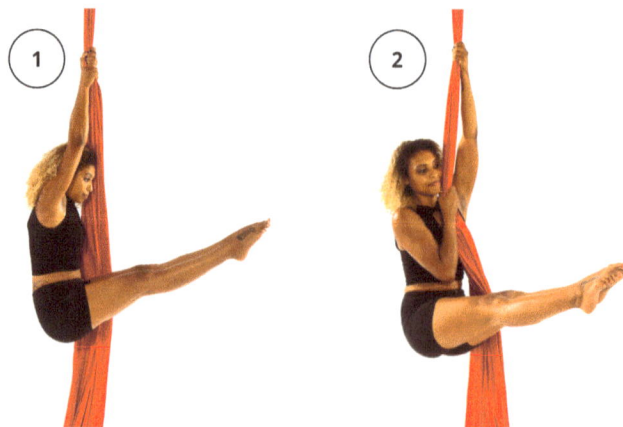

OBLIQUE CRUNCH

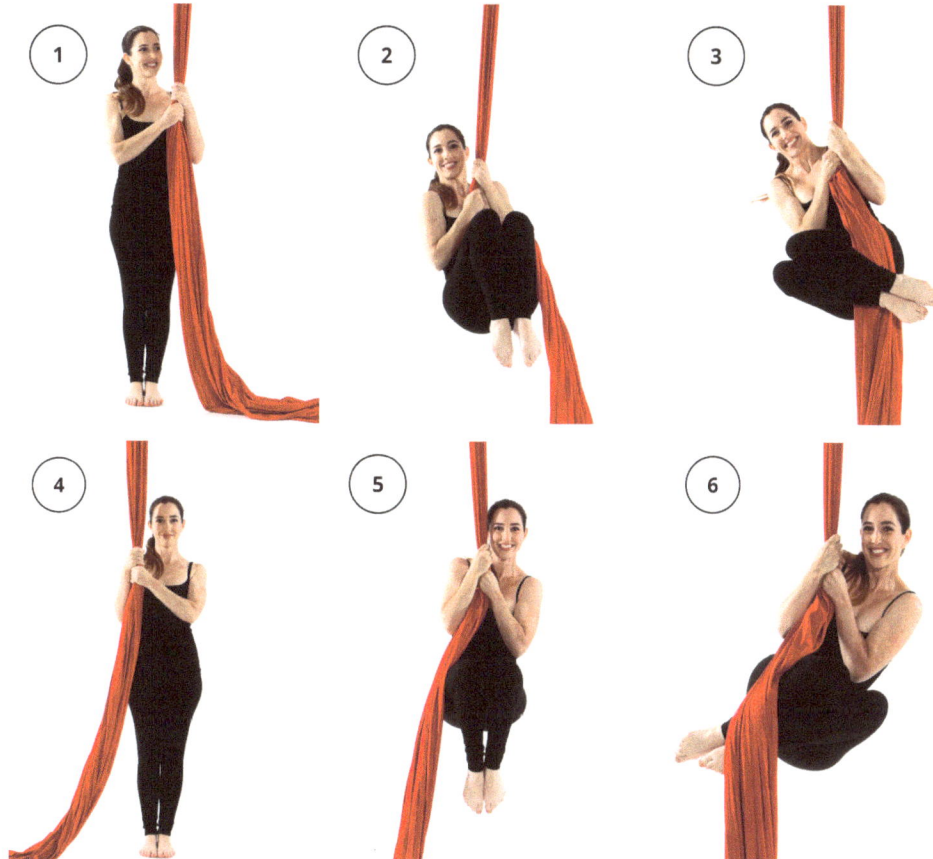

To begin, grab the fabric around or above shoulder height. Glue your legs together, feet together, and pull your navel into your spine. Hold onto the fabric and pull your body up with your hands into your heart. Make sure to use your latissimus dorsi muscle to pull your shoulders down and back. With your hands in front of your chest, bring your legs into a tuck position. Next, lift your right hip up into the air doing a side crunch, so your hips become parallel to the ground. Do 1 set of 10, then repeat to the other side.

CLIMBING PROGRESSION

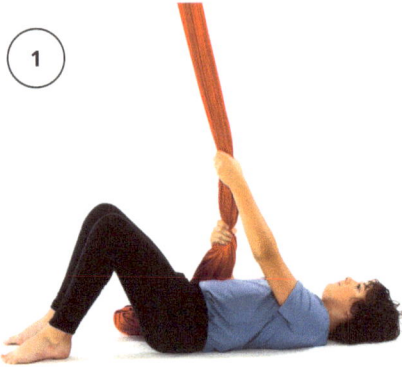

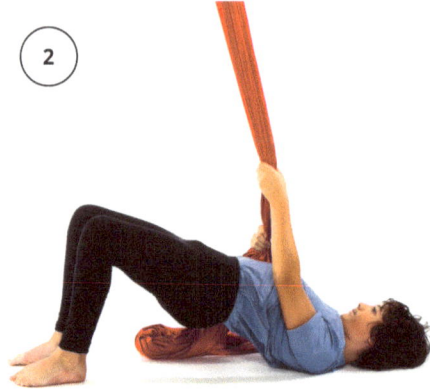

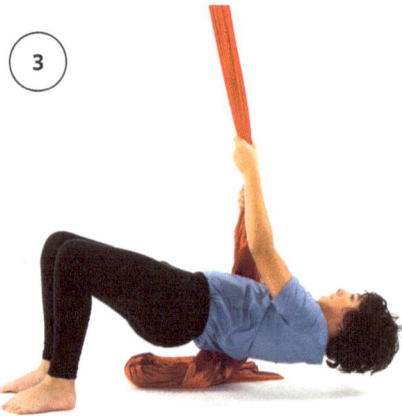

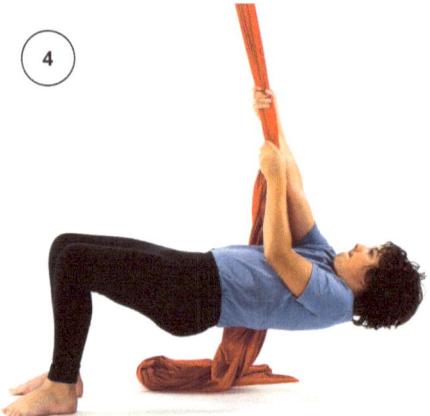

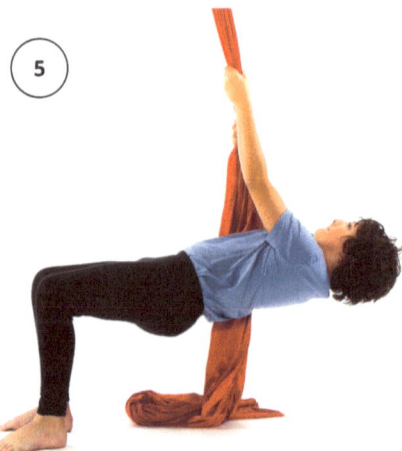

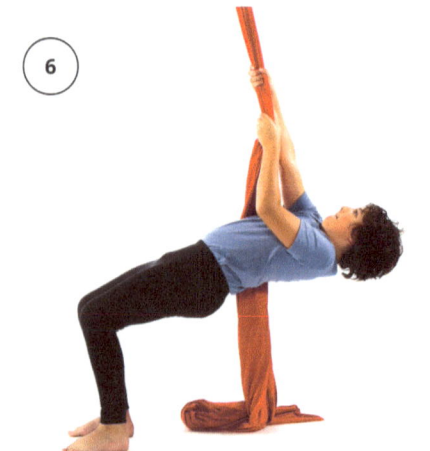

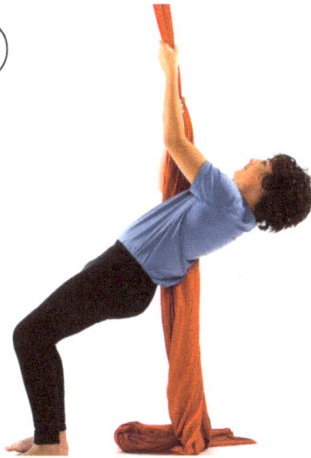

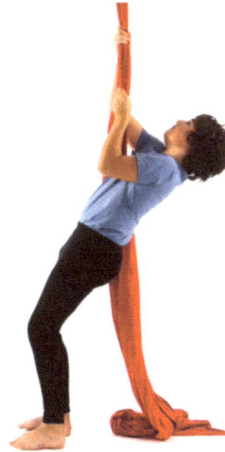

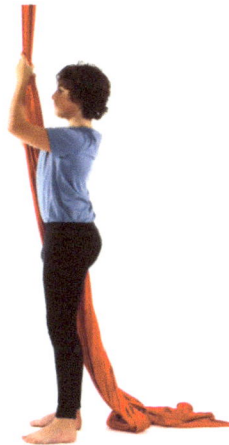

To begin, lay down on your back with the fabric on one side of your body. Bend your knees with your feet on the ground. Shoot your hips up into the air, engage your core muscles, and try to maintain this position throughout this exercise. Walk your hands up the fabric hand over hand until you are standing up straight. Next, start to walk your hands down the fabric hand over hand. Bend your knees as you are going down and continue to shoot your hips up to create a straight position in your upper body. Use your legs to help you stand up and down until you build strength in your arms. Do 1 set of 10.

As you gain strength, be sure to rely more on your arm strength to pull yourself up the fabric.

AERIAL SILK CLIMB

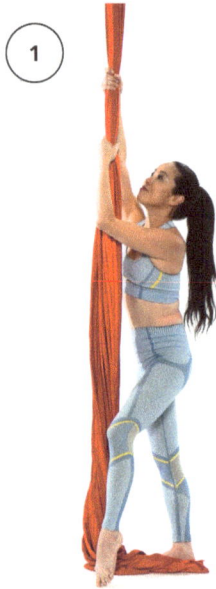

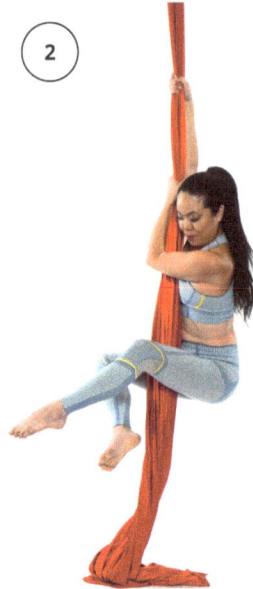

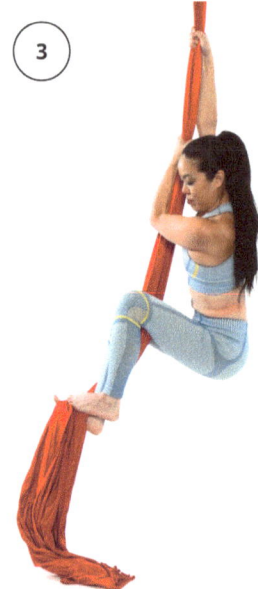

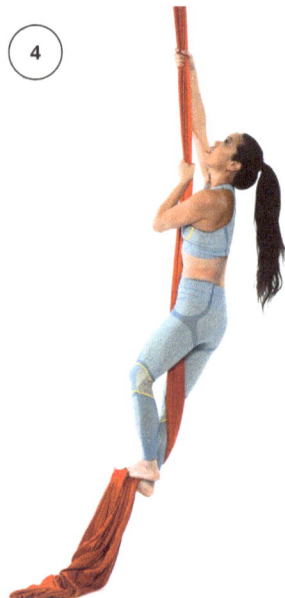

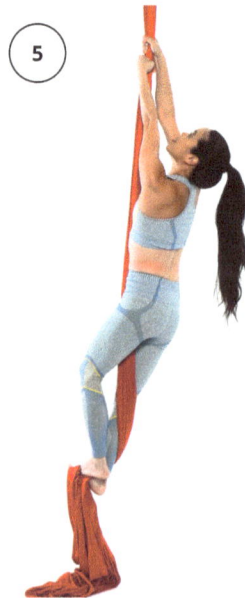

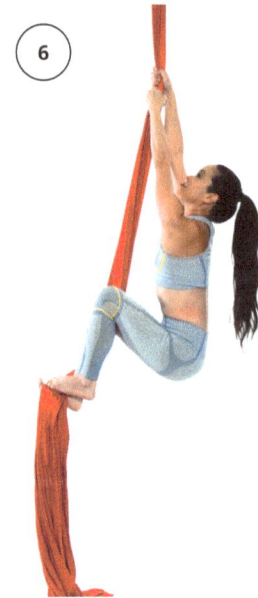

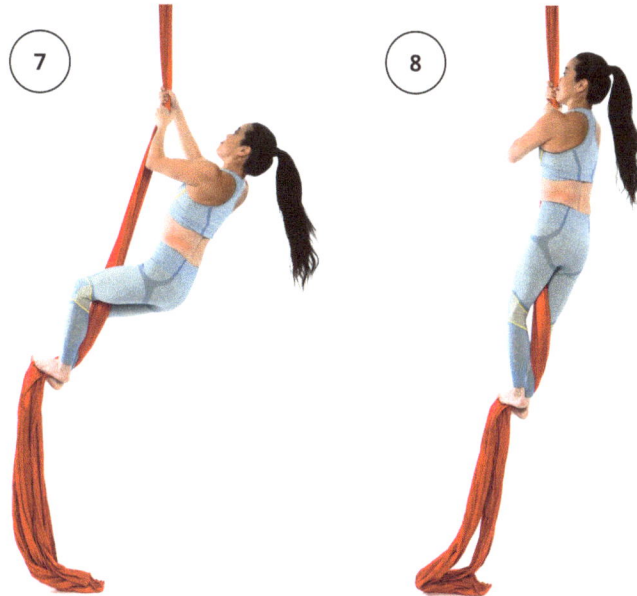

To begin, face the fabric and center it to your body. Grab the fabric above your head with both hands. Similar to a tuck crunch, pull your knees toward your chest while wrapping the fabric like you are hugging it with your leg. Then immediately step on both the top of the fabric and the other foot with your free foot. Use your legs to help you stand up and your arms to pull your body up the fabric until you are in a standing position. **Always remember to keep the wrapped foot flexed so the fabric will not slip off.** Walk your arms up the fabric and repeat all the steps until you reach your desired height or the top of the fabric. Do 3–5 climbs on each side.

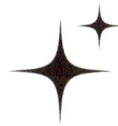

PRO TIP: ONLY GO TO THE HEIGHT THAT YOU FEEL SAFE AND MAKE SURE YOU HAVE ENOUGH ENERGY TO COME DOWN SAFELY

AERIAL SILK CLIMB DESCEND

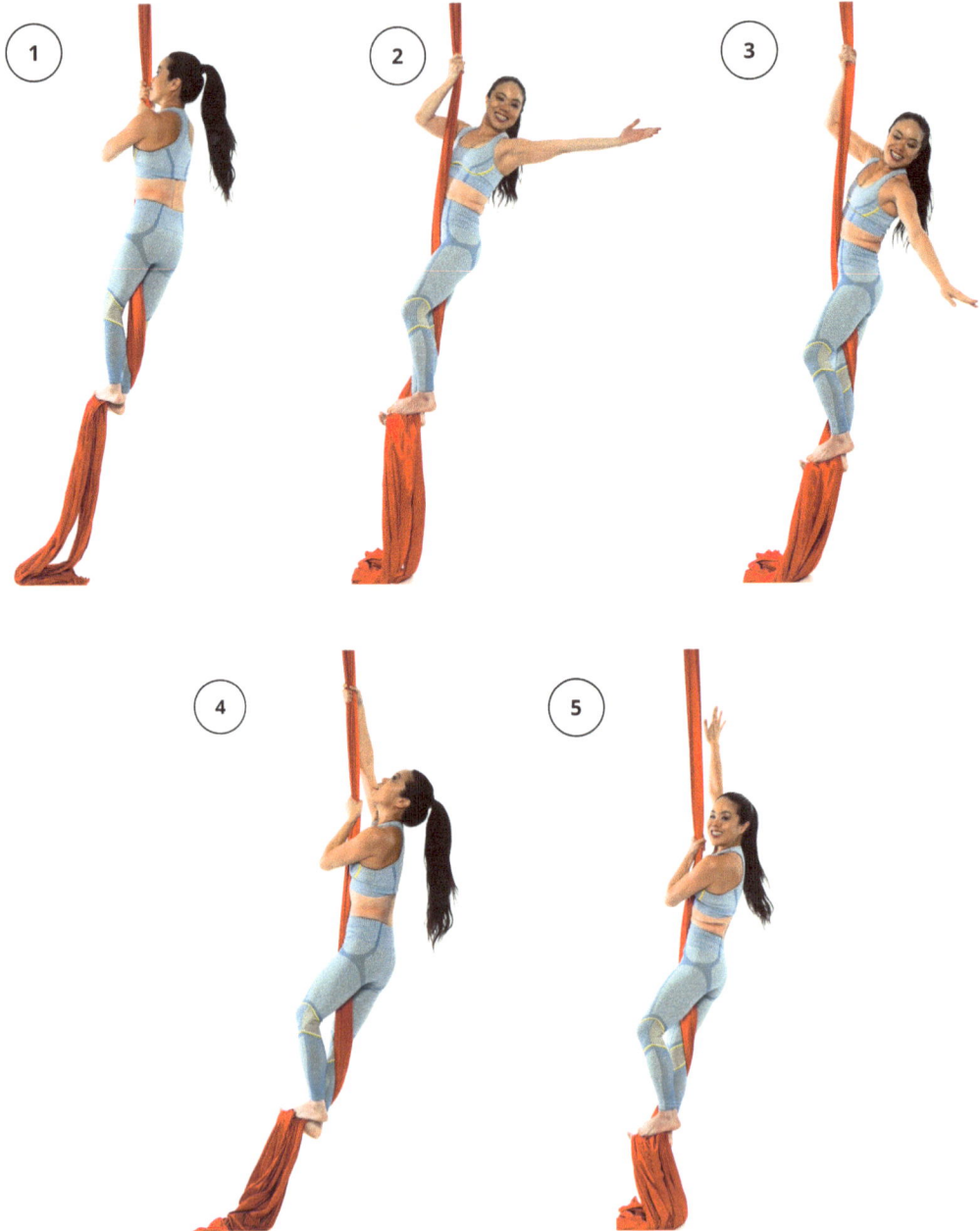

After you climb to the top of the fabric, hold the fabric with your hands at about chest level. Slowly release tension in your top foot to allow the fabric to glide between your feet as you descend. **Never remove your top foot from the fabric.** Slide down the fabric hand over hand until you return to the ground.

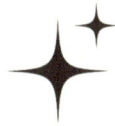

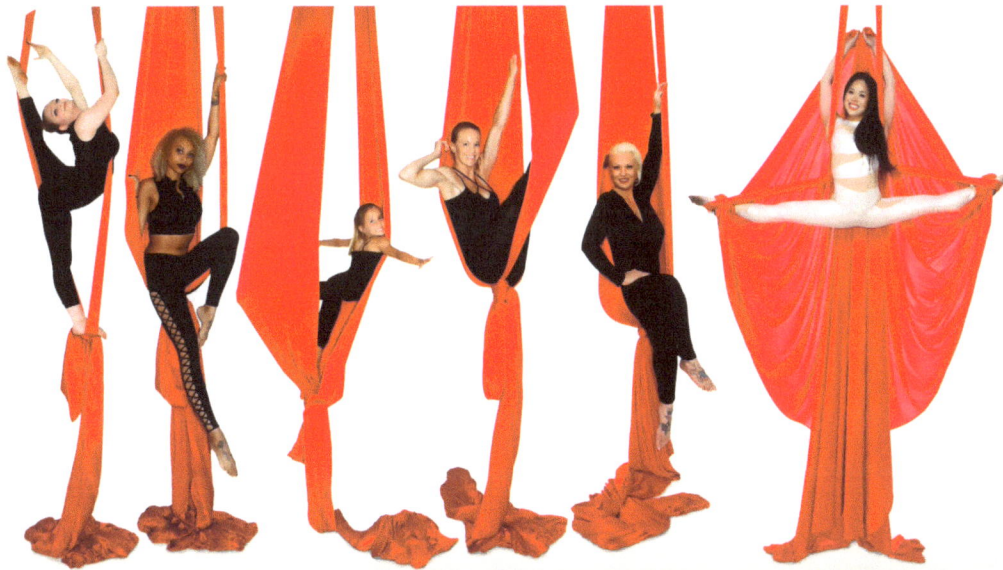

ASSISTED PIKE DESCEND

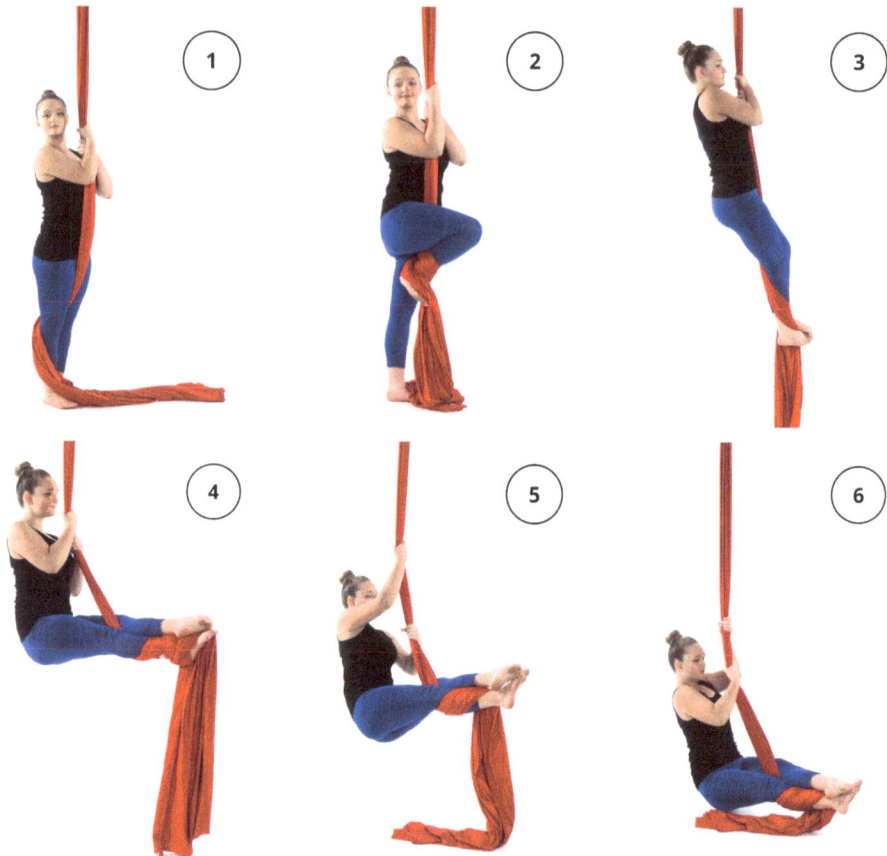

To begin, do a single-leg wrap on the aerial silk. Grab the fabric around or above shoulder height. Glue your legs together, feet together, and pull your navel into your spine. Hold onto the fabric and lift the wrapped leg into a tuck position. Pull your body up with your hands into your heart. Make sure to use your latissimus dorsi muscle to pull your shoulders down and back. Step your unwrapped foot on top of your other foot. Extend your legs forward into an "L" sit or a 90° pike position. For additional support, cross your free leg over the other leg. Make sure to keep the fabric wrapped around your leg to let it assist and support you. Move down the fabric hand over hand with your legs in the pike position until you return to the ground.

PIKE DESCEND

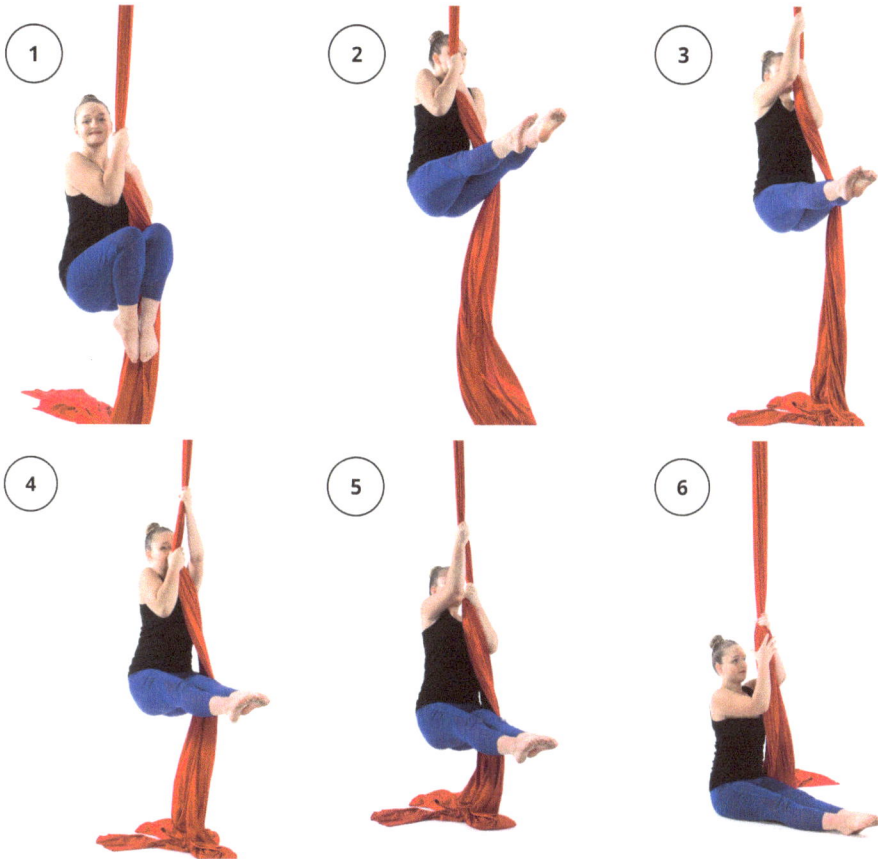

To begin, grab the fabric around or above shoulder height. Glue your legs together, feet together, and pull your navel into your spine. Hold onto the fabric and pull your body up with your hands into your heart. Make sure to use your latissimus dorsi muscle to pull your shoulders down and back. From a tuck position, extend your legs forward into an "L" sit or a 90° pike position. Walk down the fabric hand over hand with your legs in the pike position until you return to the ground.

PIKE CLIMB

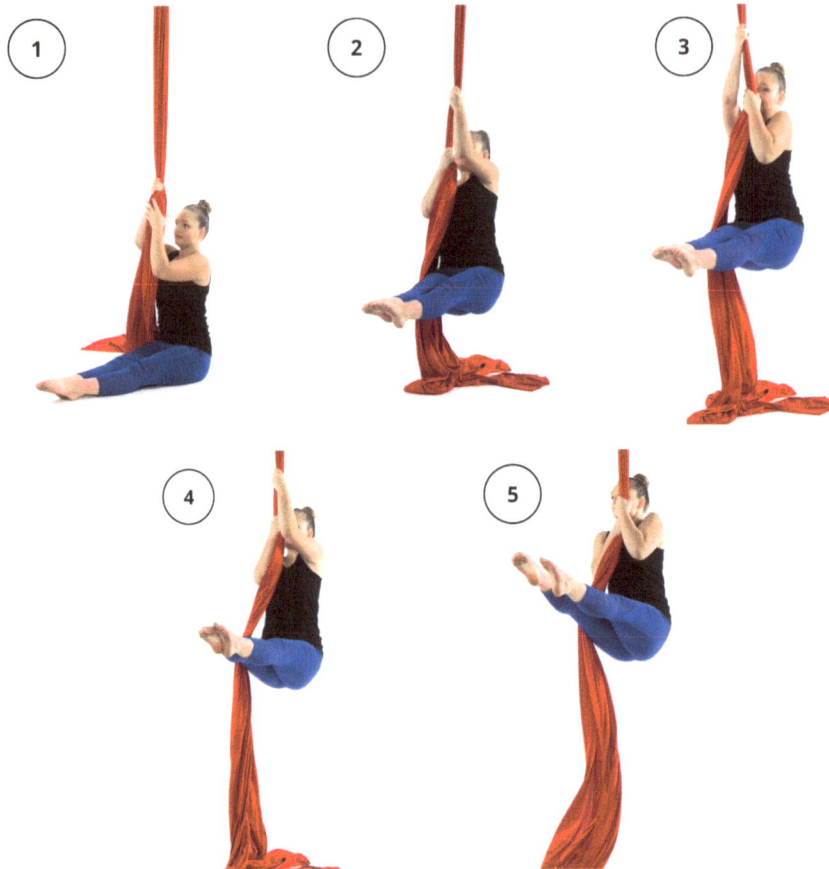

First, sit on the ground in a pike position with the fabric at your right or left hip. Grab the fabric around shoulder height. Maintain your pike position throughout this exercise. Hold onto the fabric and pull your body up with your hands into your heart. Make sure to use your latissimus dorsi muscle to pull your shoulders down and back. Move up the fabric hand over hand as high as you can go. Put your legs down to stand up when you need to. Repeat with the fabric at the other hip.

STRADDLE LEG LIFTS

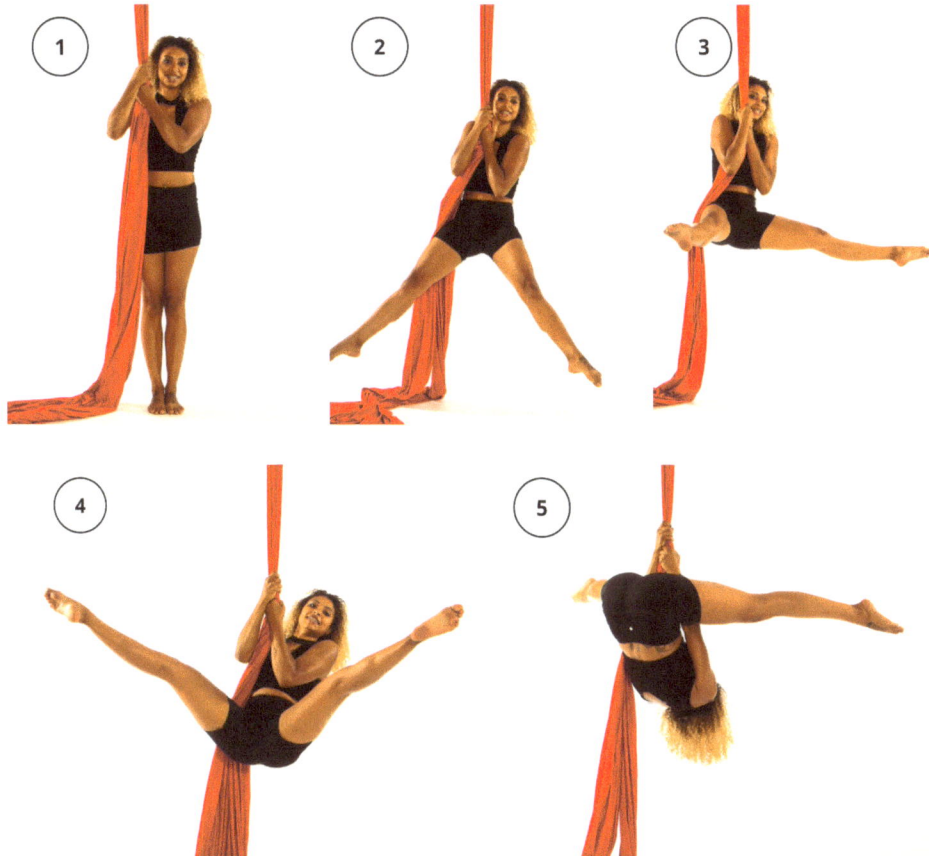

To begin, grab the fabric around or above shoulder height. Glue your legs together, feet together, and pull your navel into your spine. Hold onto the fabric. Make sure to use your latissimus dorsi muscle to pull your shoulders down and back. Pull your body up with your hands in front of your heart. Keep both legs straight as you move through the straddle position, and extend your arms as you invert your body. Then move your legs back down through the straddle position, and bend your arms to bring your hands back to your heart. Do 1 set of 10.

Aerial Fitness Goals

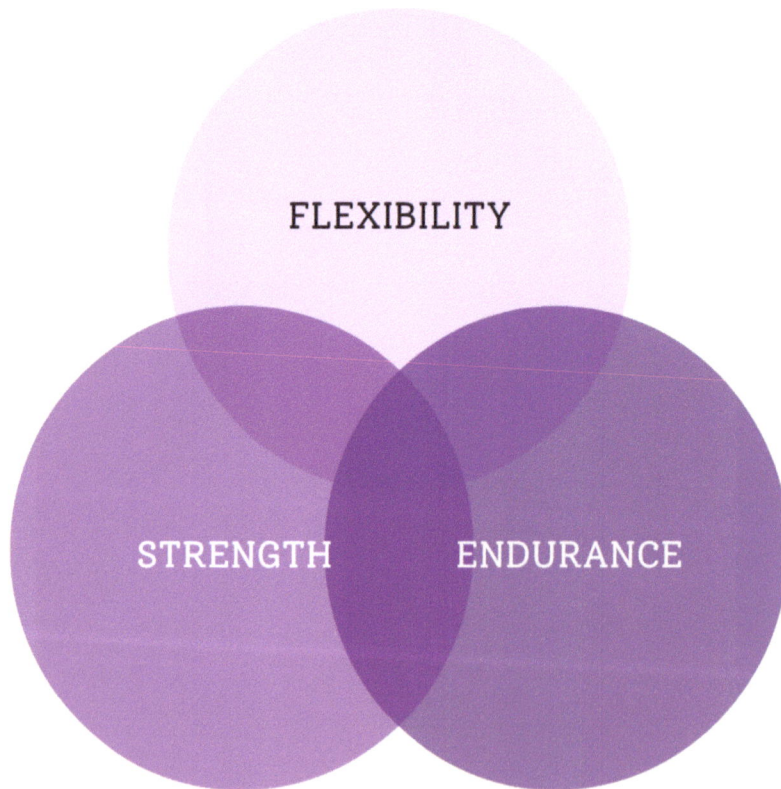

FLEXIBILITY

STRENGTH   ENDURANCE

Build your strength, increase your flexibility, and gain endurance.

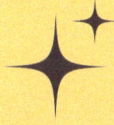

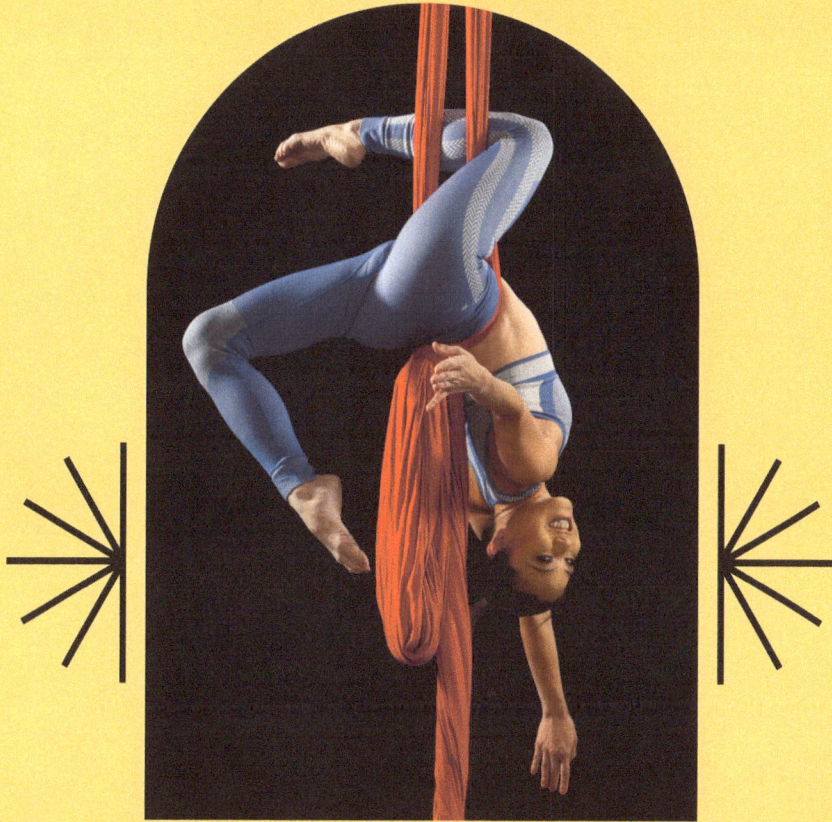

AERIAL FITNESS

HAMMOCK KNOT

A hammock knot is similar to a slip knot in the crochet technique, except the arm is the needle and the fabric is the yarn.

How To Tie A Hammock Knot

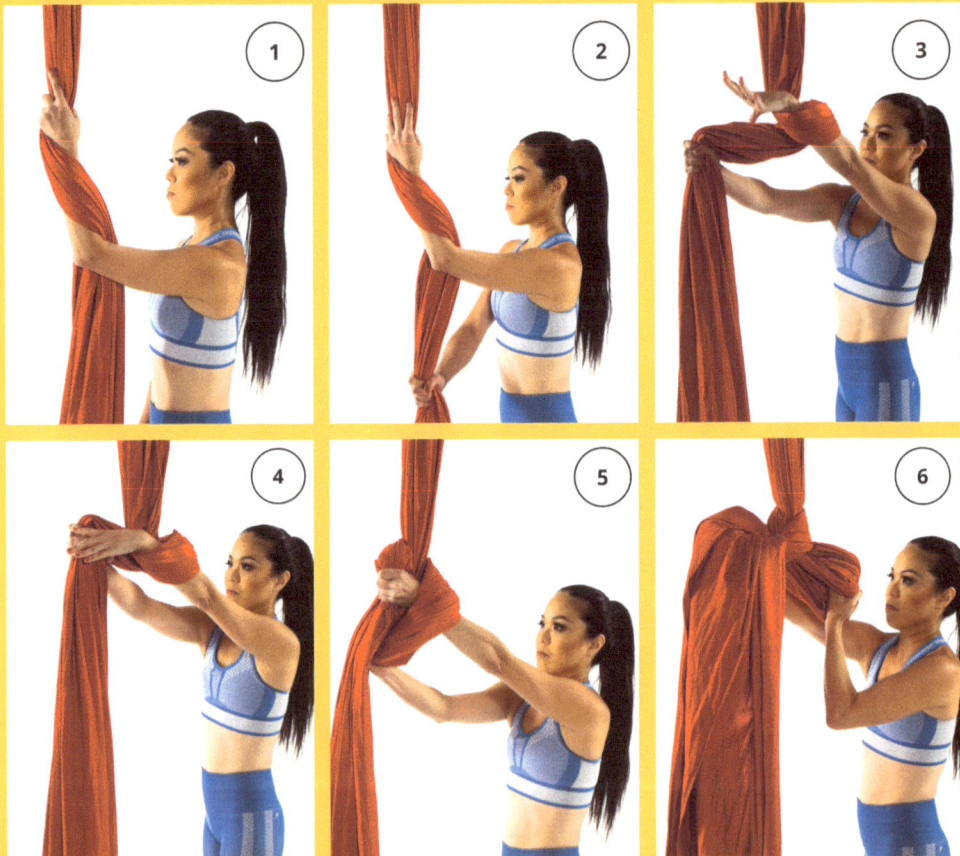

First, wrap the fabric around your arm like you are hugging the fabric with your hand heading up into the air. Pick up the dangling fabric with the opposite hand about 1 foot below the other hand. Then place the fabric into the higher hand and pull your hand through the hole that is made holding on to the fabric. Pull the fabric down tight to cinch the knot. Ensure there is significant slack beneath the knot so it will not untie on accident. To undo the knot, pull the tail of the fabric until the knot disappears.

GOOD KNOT

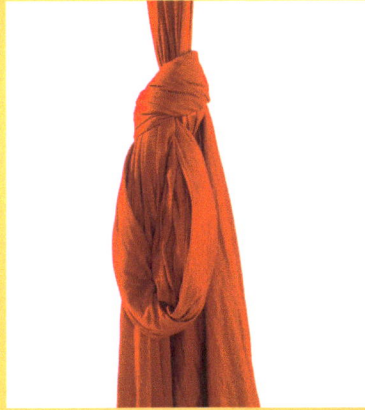

Long loop below knot

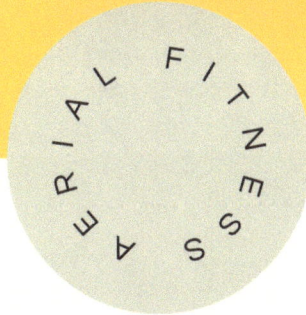

AERIAL FITNESS

BAD KNOT

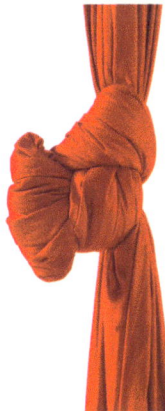

Short loop below knot

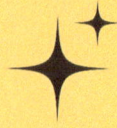

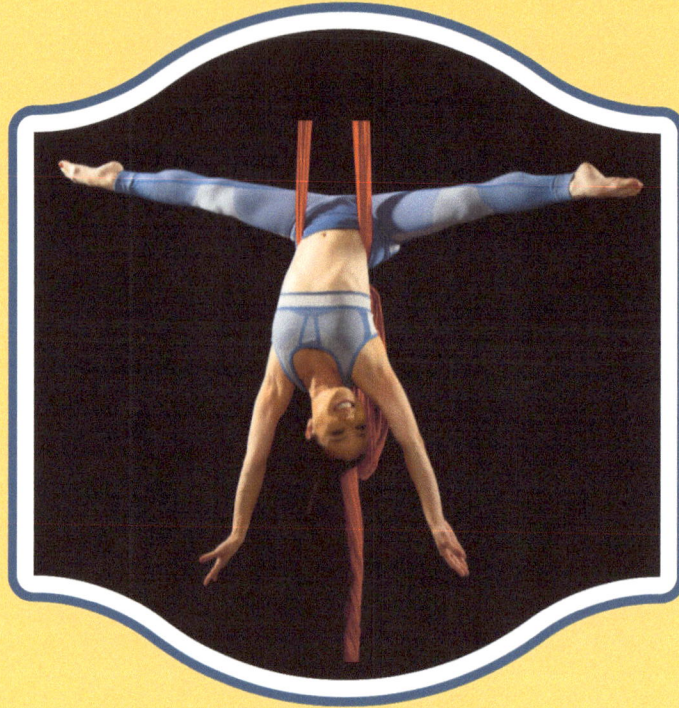

AERIAL FITNESS

HAMMOCK KNOT TECHNIQUE

The hammock knot is a great knot that will allow beginners to have assistance to explore more range of movement on the aerial silk.

89

HAMMOCK KNOT SIT-UPS

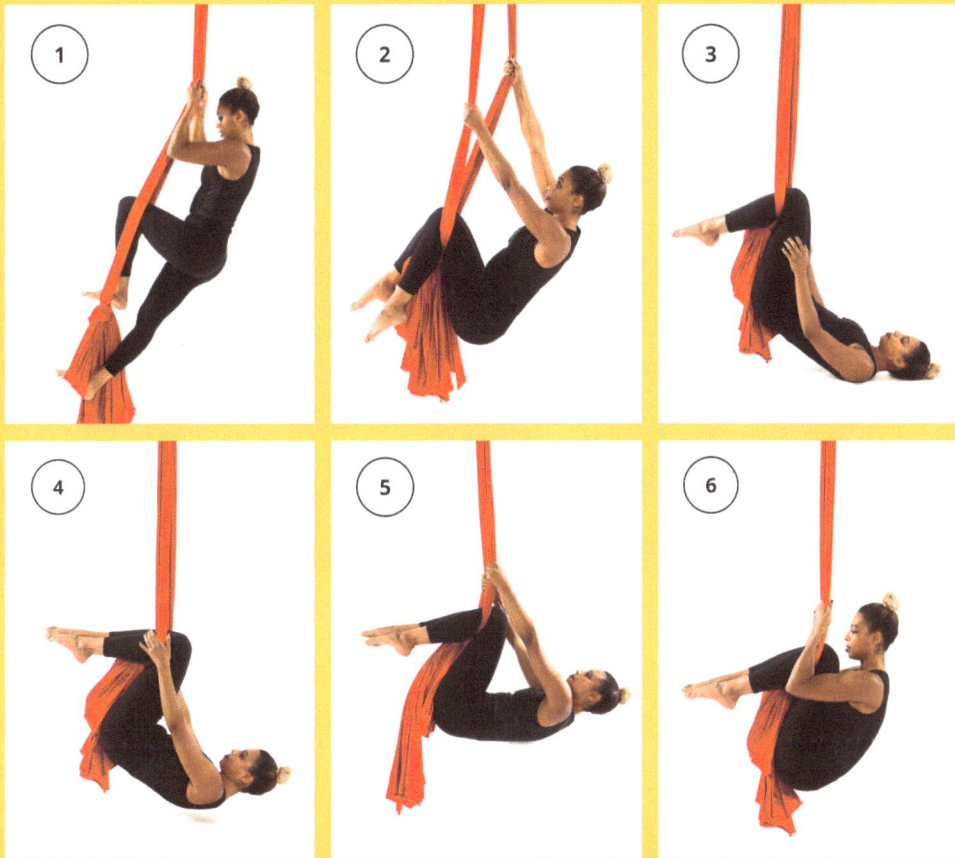

To begin, tie a hammock knot. You can use the loop created below the knot as a step. Sit in the swing made above the knot. Hold onto both sides of the fabric and slowly lower your body to the ground with your knees bent to catch the fabric behind your knees. Use caution, as your head may touch the ground. You may feel pressure behind your knees, so adjust your position as needed. If it is too much pressure on your knees, stop and come down safely. Once hanging from your knees in a good position, kick your feet toward the ground to create more safety. Next, sit up and place your head on your knees. If this is difficult, you can safely grab your legs or the fabric above the knot to help you sit up. Then safely lower your body back to the ground. Start low to the ground until you gain the strength to hang without your head on the ground. Do 1 set of 10-20.

HAMMOCK KNOT FOOT HANG SIT-UPS

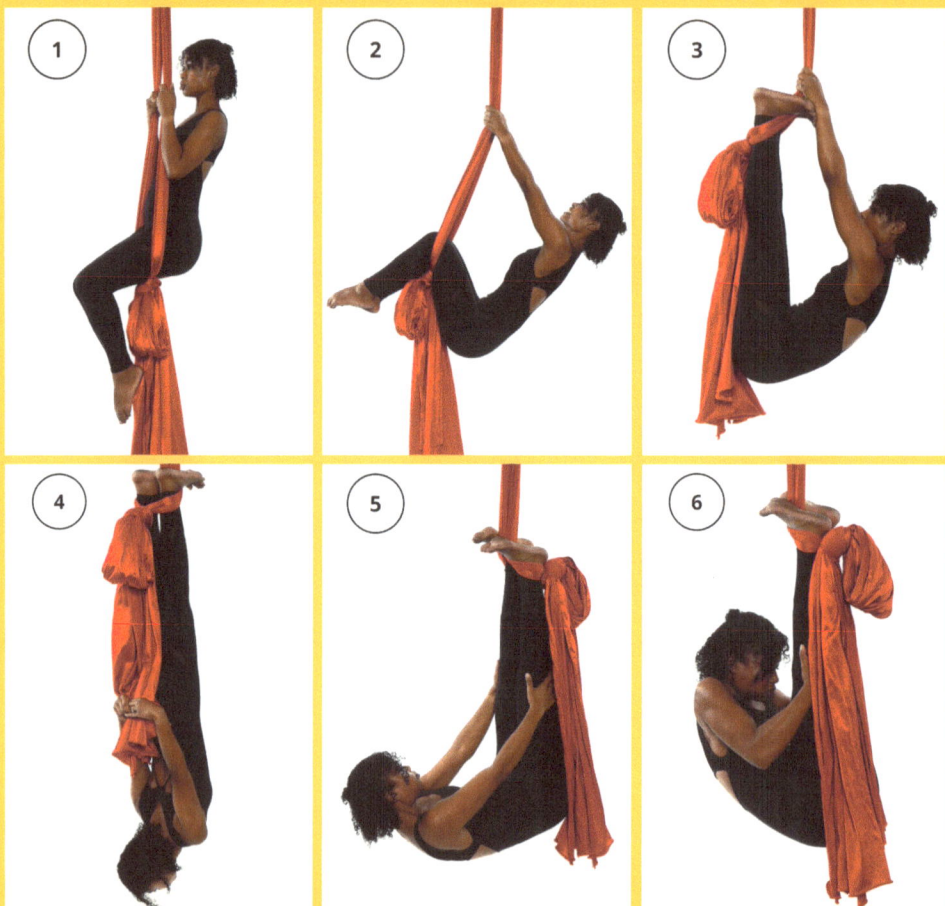

To begin, tie a hammock knot. You can use the loop created below the knot as a step. Start in the Hammock Knot Sit-Up position. Hold onto both sides of the fabric and slowly slide the fabric to your feet as you lower your body to the ground. Be careful as your head may touch the ground. You may feel pressure on your ankles or feet, so adjust as needed. If it is too much pressure on your ankles or feet, stop and come down safely. **Make sure to flex your feet to make sure you don't slip out of the fabric.** Then, sit up and try to place your head on your knees. If this is too difficult, you can use your arms to grab behind your legs to help you sit up. Then safely lower your body back to the ground. Do 1 set of 10-20.

91

HAMMOCK KNOT LEG DROP

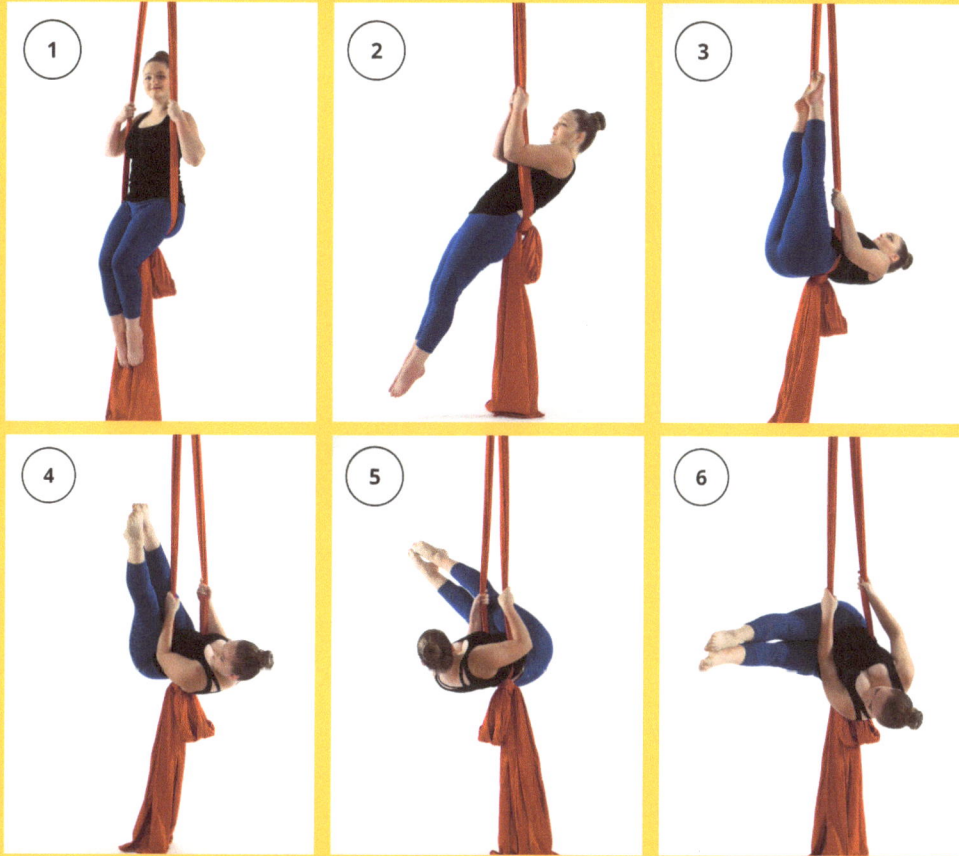

To begin, tie a hammock knot. Sit in the hammock knot swing. Hold onto the fabric and lean back in a pike position with your back parallel to the ground, and your feet shooting up into the air. Keep your legs straight and slowly lower your legs to the right and try to keep your back parallel to the ground. Next, lift your legs back up and lower your legs down to the left, then lift your legs back up to the center position. If it is too difficult to straighten your legs, try this exercise with bent legs until you build the strength to straighten your legs. Do 1 set of 10.

HAMMOCK KNOT PLANK

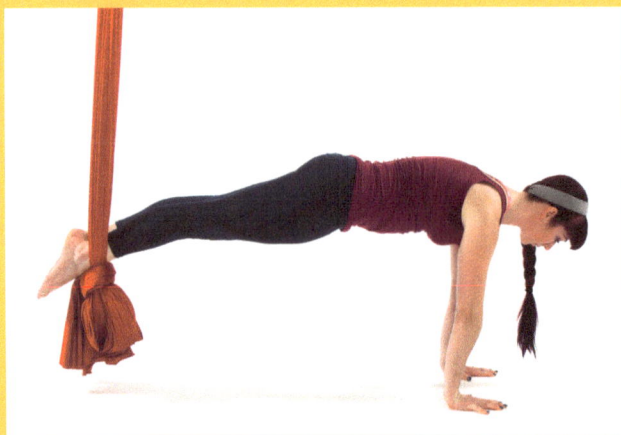

To begin, tie the hammock knot so you can comfortably be in a plank position. Place the top of your feet onto the hammock knot with your body parallel to the ground. The palms of your hands should be flat on the ground with your arms fully extended. Hold the position for 20, 30, or 60 seconds.

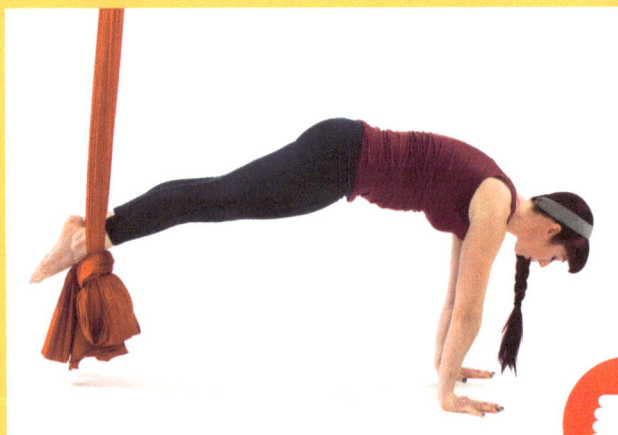

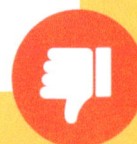

TECHNIQUE TIP: DO NOT SHOOT YOUR HIPS UP INTO THE AIR. LOWER YOUR HIPS AND ENGAGE YOUR CORE TO CREATE A FLAT BACK

HAMMOCK KNOT PLANK TUCK

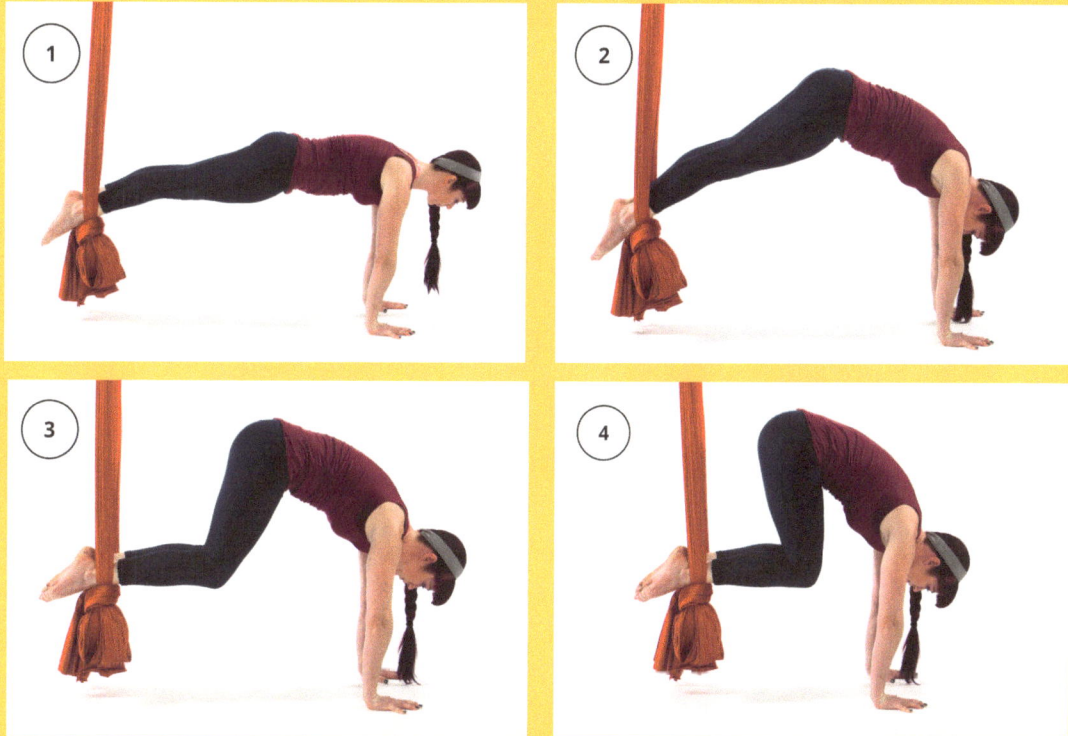

To begin, tie the hammock knot so you can comfortably be in a plank position. Place the top of your feet onto the hammock knot with your body parallel to the ground. The palms of your hand should be flat on the ground with your arms fully extended. Once you are in the Hammock Knot Plank position, pull your knees into your chest, then extend back out to the Hammock Knot Plank position. Do 1 set of 10.

✦

**PRO TIP: ENGAGE YOUR CORE TO HELP YOU
NOT BEND IN YOUR BACK
AND MAINTAIN A CORRECT POSITION**

HAMMOCK KNOT PLANK PIKE

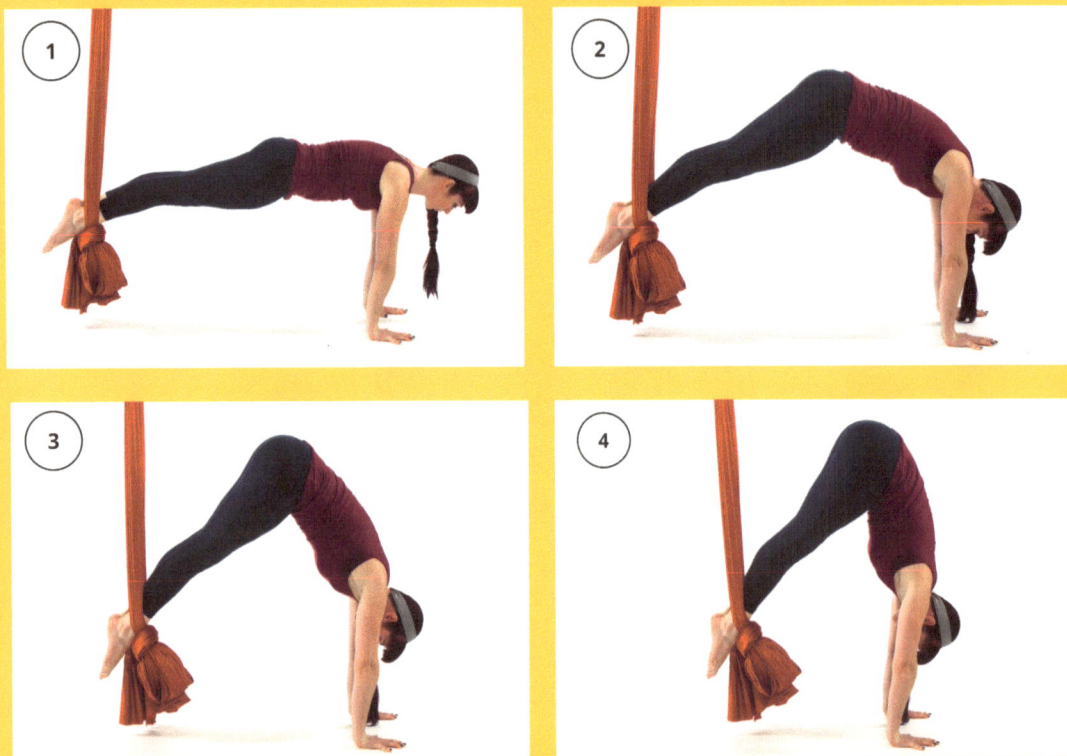

To begin, tie the hammock knot so you can comfortably be in a plank position. Place the top of your feet onto the hammock knot with your body parallel to the ground. The palms of your hand should be flat on the ground with your arms fully extended. Once in the Hammock Knot Plank position, pull your hips above your head and shoulders, then extend back out to the Hammock Knot Plank position. Do 1 set of 10.

HAMMOCK KNOT SPLITS

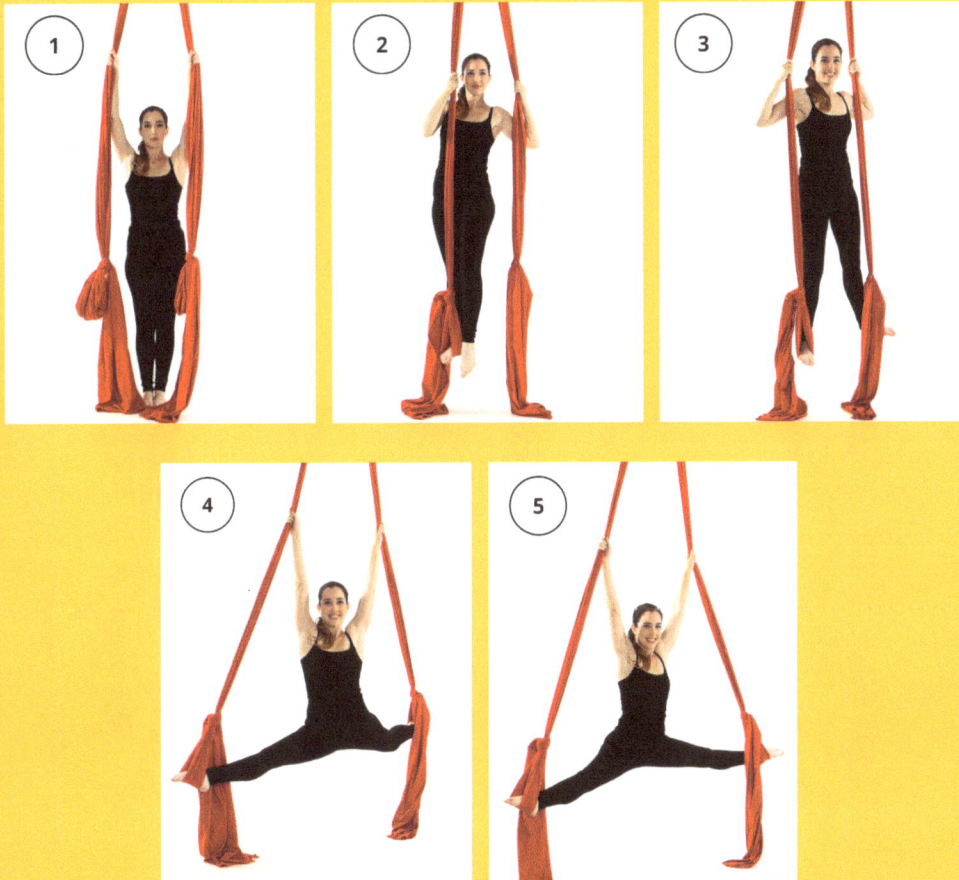

To begin, tie a hammock knot on each fabric at the same height. Hold onto each fabric separately and step into each hammock step loop created. Slowly open to your left split and hold for 10 seconds. Stand up. Repeat to the right split and center split.

HAMMOCK KNOT BACKBEND

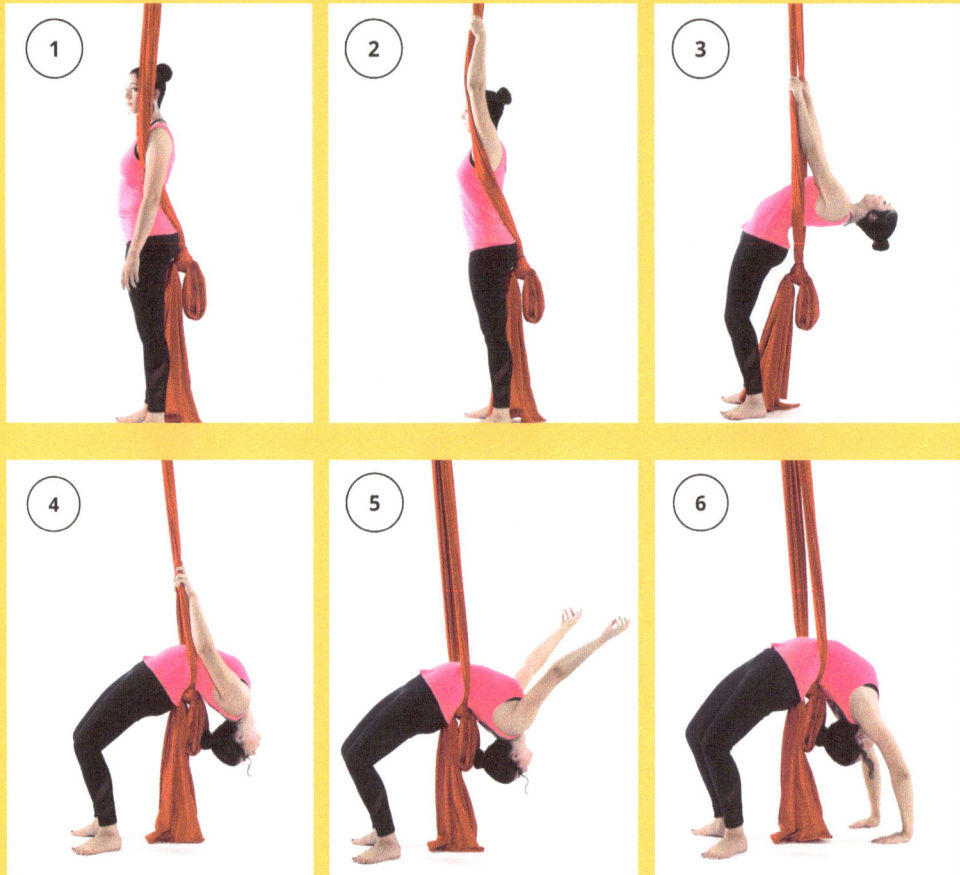

To begin, tie the hammock knot at about hip level. With the fabric behind you, place your arms through the swing and hold onto the fabric. Slowly lower yourself into a backbend with the fabric placed in your lower back. For additional support, you can continue to hold onto the fabric or let go of the fabric one hand at a time. Once you are in a bridge position, hold for 20–30 seconds or as long as desired. Then slowly and safely grab the fabric if you let go to help you stand up.

Hammock Knot Cocoon

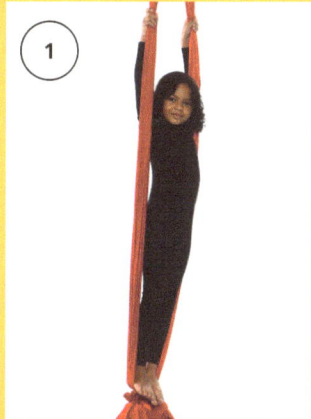

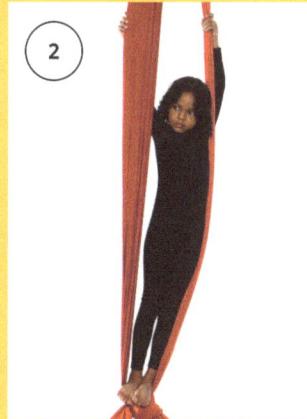

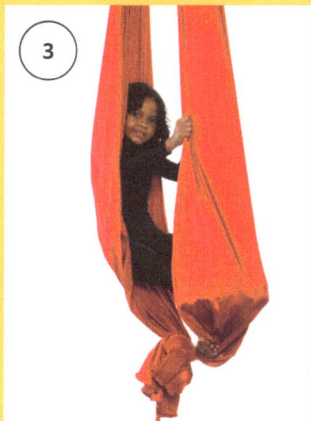

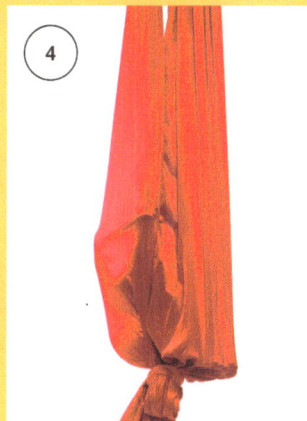

To begin, tie the hammock knot a little above the ground. Stand in the center of the hammock, then turn your body to face one side. Hold onto the fabric in front of you with one hand, then reach your other hand to grab an edge of the fabric behind you. Start to open the fabric behind you and begin to sit down in the fabric. As you continue to get into a seated position, start to open up the fabric in front of you. Place your feet into the fabric in front of you and bend your knees into a tuck position and sit down. Bring together the edges of both sides of the fabric and enclose your body in the fabric.

Hammock Knot Cocoon Plank

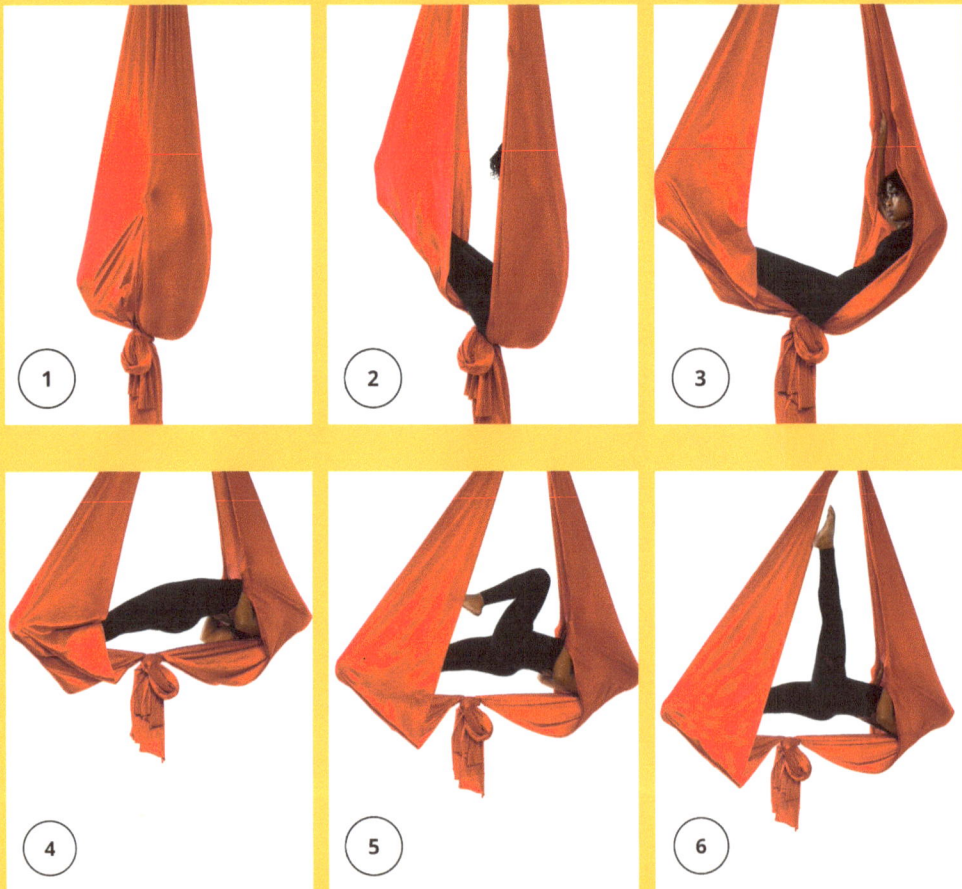

To begin, tie the hammock knot a little above the ground. Start in a Hammock Knot Cocoon position. Lift both hands straight up into the air and grab the edges of the fabric behind you. Begin to straighten your legs and extend your feet up the front piece of fabric. Start to pull up with your arms and shoot your hips up into the air. Remember to lengthen your spine to the crown of your head. For more of a challenge, extend one leg straight up into the air.

Hammock Knot Sailboat

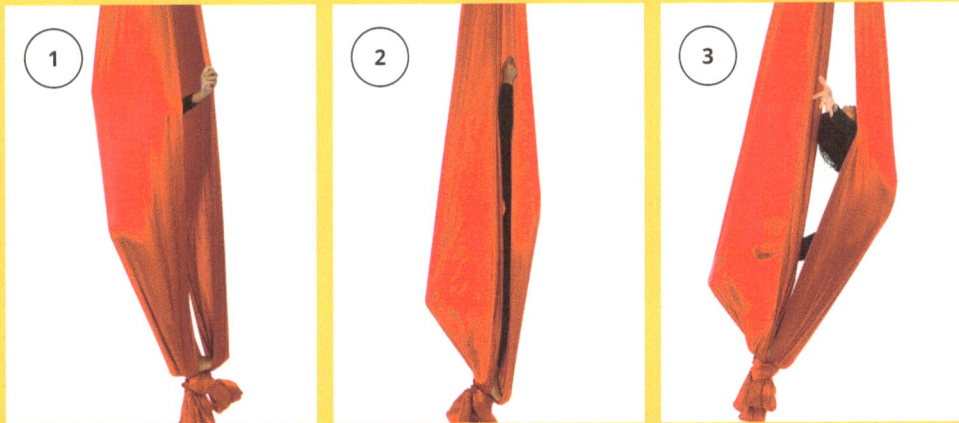

To begin, tie the hammock knot a little above the ground. Start in the Hammock Knot Cocoon position and stand up by pressing your back into the fabric behind you. Place one foot in front of the knot and one foot behind the knot and hold onto the edges of the front piece of fabric. Begin to shift your whole body to the fabric in front of you by pressing your chest into the front piece of fabric. Then, back kick or arabesque one leg into the open fabric behind you. Once you feel safe, let go of the fabric and extend your arms to the side and look back.

✦

PRO TIP: TO GET YOUR BACK LEG HIGHER, POINT YOUR FOOT AND GLIDE THE TOP OF YOUR FOOT UP THE FABRIC

✦

HAMMOCK KNOT ANGEL

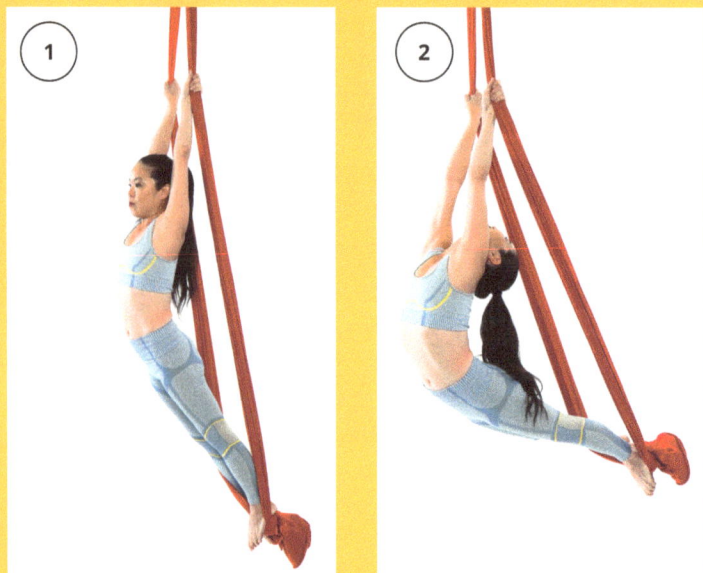

To begin, tie the hammock knot at about hip level or higher. Stand in the center of the fabric holding onto both sides with your hands above your head. Move your shoulders in front of the fabric and begin to slide your hands down the fabric. Arch your back and look back. To easily return to the center of the fabric, bend both knees, then return to a standing position.

PRO TIP: MOVE YOUR FREE LEG INTO PASSÉ POSITION, THEN EXTEND INTO A SPLIT POSITION TO CREATE DIFFERENT SHAPES

HAMMOCK KNOT SUPERMAN

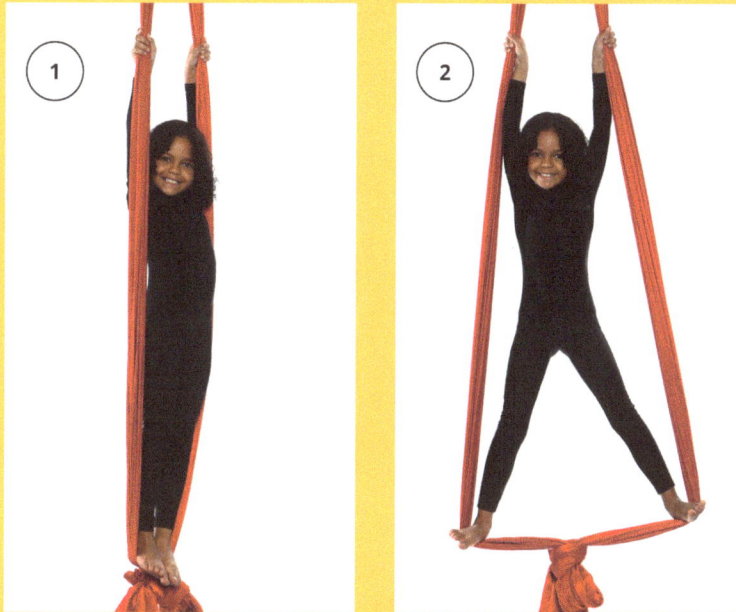

To begin, tie the hammock knot a little above the ground. Stand in the center of the fabric grabbing both sides of the fabric with your arms fully extended. Step up on one side of the fabric at a time, then stand up.

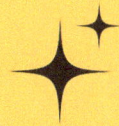

**PRO TIP: ENGAGE YOUR CORE FOR MORE
STABILITY IN THE AIR**

HAMMOCK KNOT BACK SPLIT

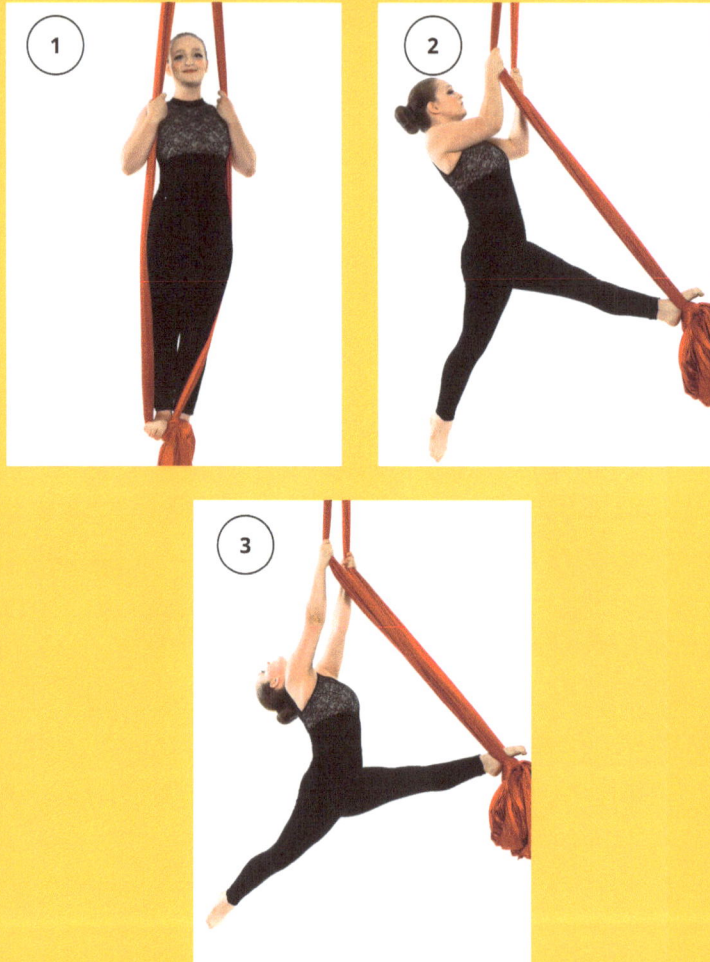

To begin, tie the hammock knot at about hip level or higher. Stand in the center of the fabric. Hold onto both sides of the fabric with your hands about chest level. Slowly extend your arms and slide your hands down a little while moving a leg in arabesque to reach a side split position. Look back. Repeat to the other side.

HAMMOCK KNOT STRADDLE INVERSION

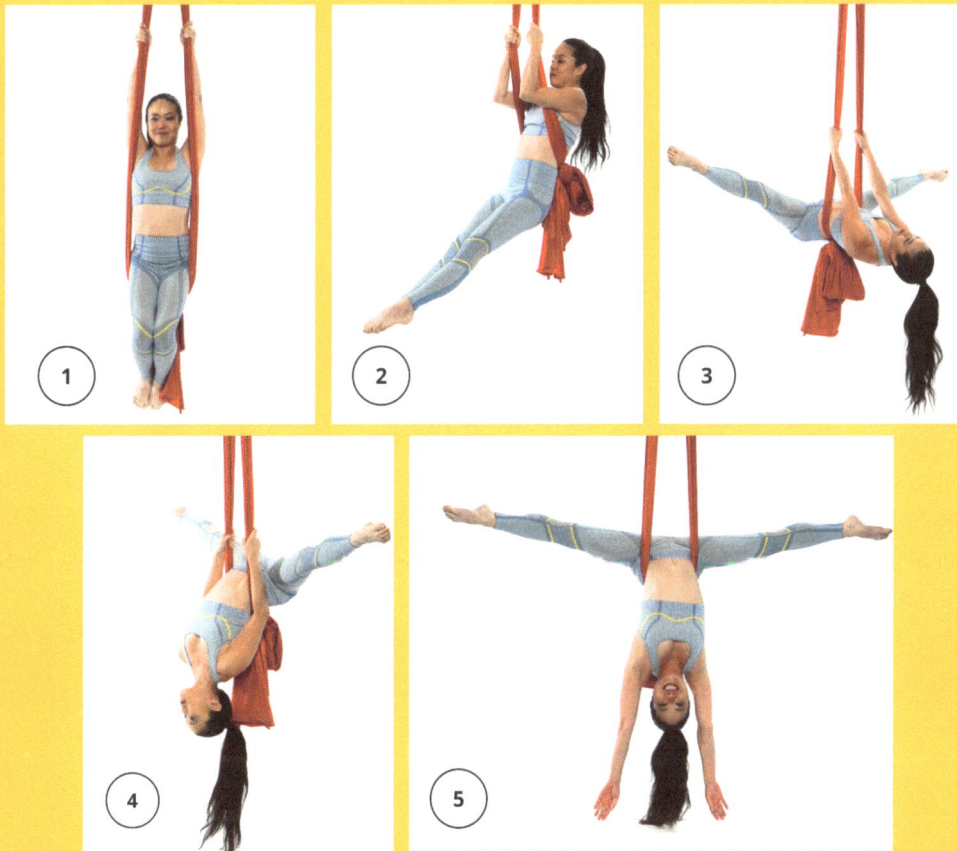

To begin, tie the hammock knot at about hip level or higher. Sit in the hammock knot like a swing. Hold onto the fabric, and slowly lower your body down the fabric so the fabric moves from under your glutes to your lower back. Once the fabric is in your lower back, start to lean back and move your leg into a straddle split position. Once you are fully inverted and feel safe, let go with both hands. Hold for 10–30 seconds.

HAMMOCK KNOT SPLIT STAG INVERSION

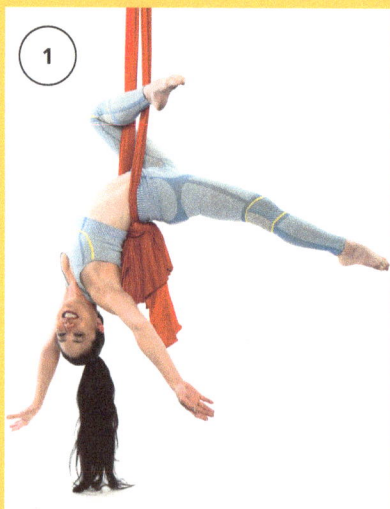

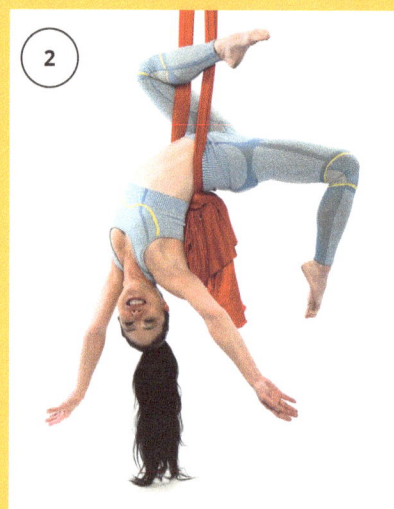

To begin, tie the hammock knot at about hip level or higher. Start in a Hammock Knot Straddle Inversion position. Bend one leg across the front of both pieces of fabric above you. Rotate your other hip to allow the other leg to move into an arabesque position, then bend the back leg. Next, straighten the back leg into an arabesque position. Then rotate that hip to allow the back leg to move back into a straddle position. Extend the other leg into a straddle position. Then repeat to the other side.

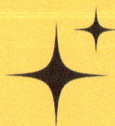

PRO TIP: GRAB YOUR FOOT FOR A DEEPER STRETCH

HAMMOCK KNOT STRADDLE INVERSION FLIP

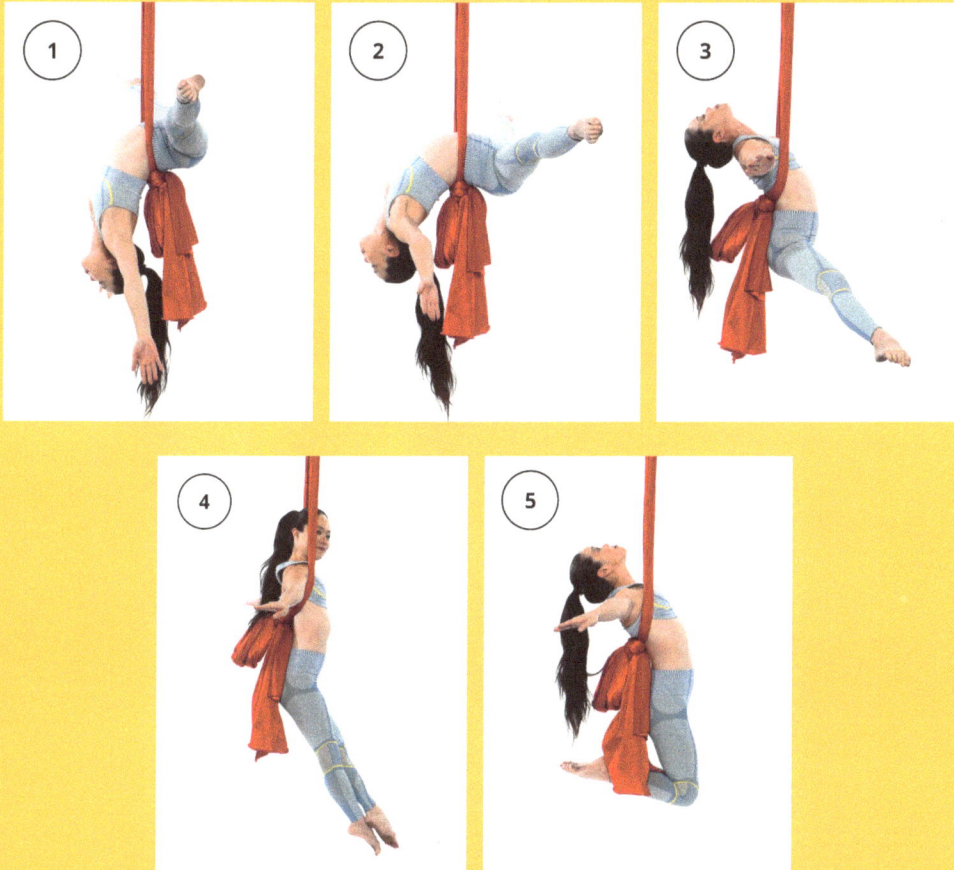

To begin, tie the hammock knot at about hip level or above. Start in a Hammock Knot Straddle Inversion position. Move your arms parallel to the ground in a "T" position. **Make sure to keep your arms in this position to ensure you don't slip through the fabric.** Start to move your legs down to the ground bringing your legs together. The fabric will catch in your armpits. Be sure to pull your shoulders down and back. Bend your legs and look back to create a different shape.

106

PRINCIPALS
OF AERIAL

- **STRENGTH**
- **GRACE**
- **EFFORTLESSNESS**
- **FLEXIBILITY**
- **DROPS**
- **WRAP**
- **FLY**
- **TWIST**
- **BEATS**
- **INVERSIONS**
- **LEVERS**

TRAINING TOOLS

PROPS THAT WILL ASSIST YOU IN VARIOUS POSITIONS AND PROGRESSIONS.

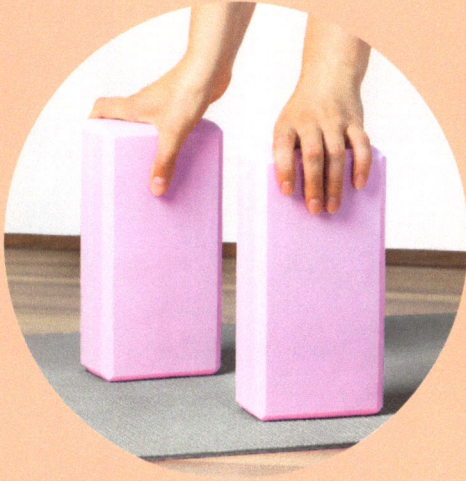

YOGA BLOCKS

Suppose you can't maintain your technique, stability, or strength to achieve the stretches being demonstrated in class. In that case, yoga blocks can help you achieve the proper position and alignment.

YOGA MAT

Your yoga mat can be a helpful tool to make sure you are always in alignment.

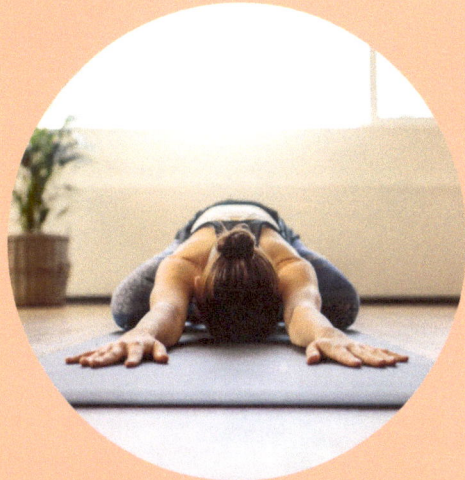

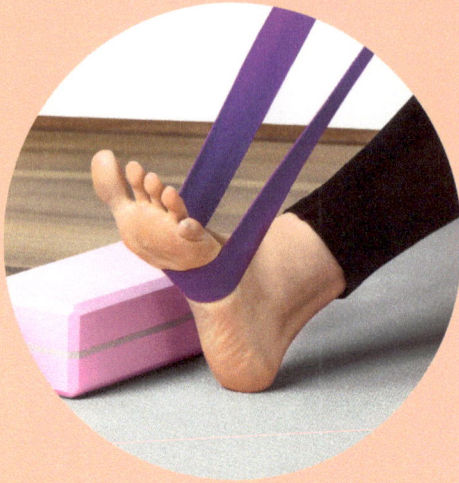

YOGA STRAP

Yoga straps may be beneficial to help you develop the flexibility to achieve different poses that seem impossible to do without assistance.

YOGA WHEEL

A yoga wheel can help you improve your flexibility by providing support to get into a deeper stretch safely.

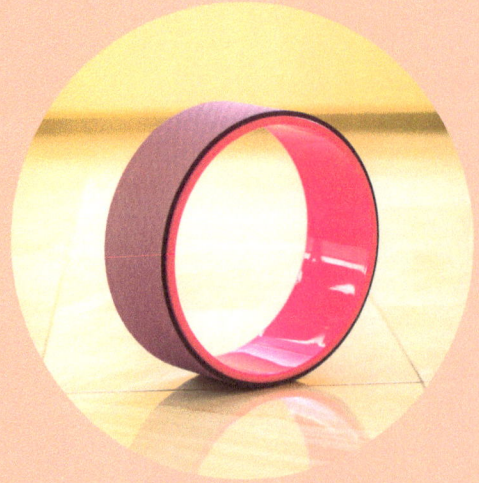

FOAM ROLLER

Foam rollers now come in all different sizes, textures, firmness, and more. You can use them before training to assist your body in your warm-up, or as post-training self-care and therapy.

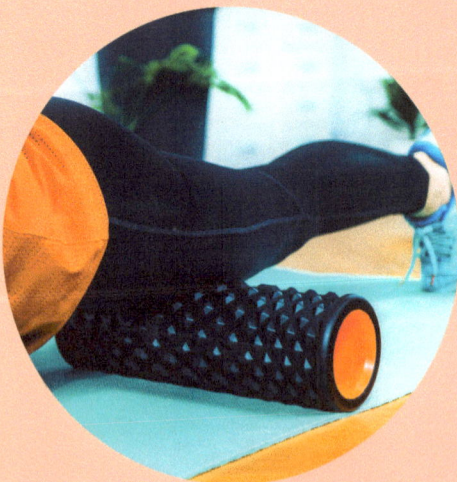

BODY RECOVERY TIPS

CREATING A SELF-CARE ROUTINE IS ESSENTIAL FOR MAINTAINING A HAPPY, HEALTHY BODY.

01

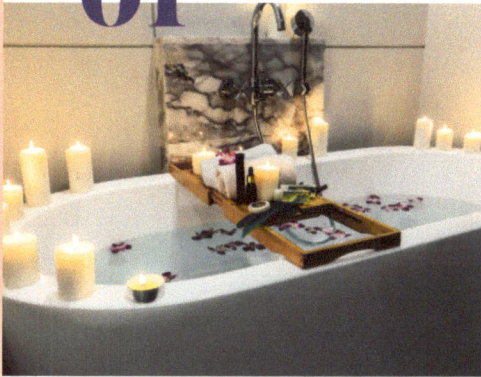

INDULGE YOURSELF

Epsom Salt Bath

Soak in 2-4 Cups of Epsom Salt in a hot bath for at least 20 minutes to aid your body, relieve pain and inflammation, and draw toxins out of your body.

02

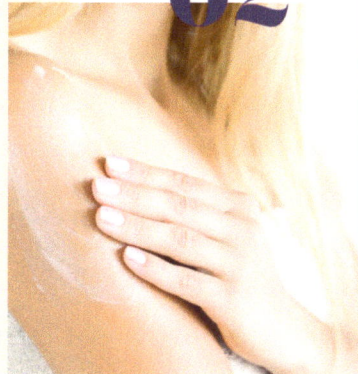

APPLY IT

Topical Treatments

Tiger Balm, Voltaren, and CBD creams are all very accessible over-the-counter topical treatments that can help you treat minor aches and pains.

03

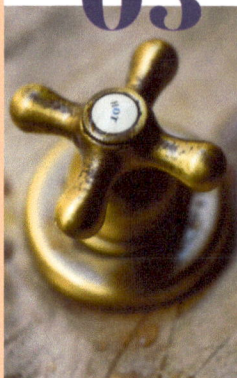

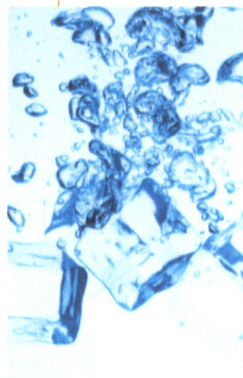

ARE YOU INJURED?

Hot/Cold Therapy

Fill a bucket or tub with the hottest water you can plunge your injured body part into where you can sit comfortably for 10-15 minutes. Then immediately plunge into an ice bath. Repeat a few times for better results.

04

USE EARTH'S GIFTS

Aromatherapy

Essential oils can help with inflammation, detoxification, and relaxation. Use Peppermint oil for muscle relief, Lemon oil for detoxification, Euculyptus oil to reduce inflammation, and Lavendar oil for relaxation.

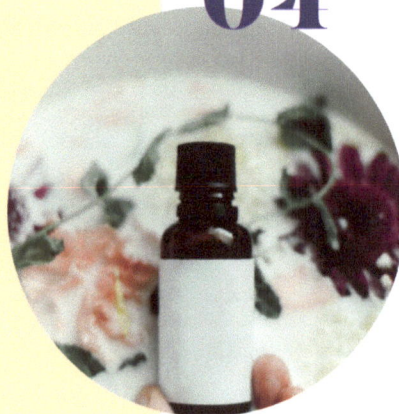

05

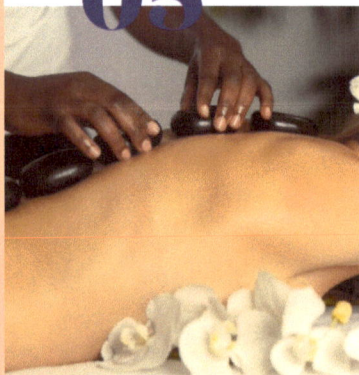

TREAT YOURSELF!

Get a Massage

Reduce your muscle tension, relieve your stress, ease your muscle pain, and increase your mobility and circulation by getting a massage. You deserve a minute for yourself to relax and breathe.

GOOD PAIN VS. BAD PAIN

At first, you may experience many foreign pains in your body. It is important to learn the difference between good and bad pain, so you can identify a possible injury in the body if it occurs.

Good pain often happens when your muscles are challenged in a new way. Although the area in pain may be sensitive to touch, the pain is temporary and will resolve in a few days.

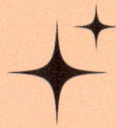

Identifying Bad Pain

- Stabbing, electric, or firey feeling
- Instant pain associated with an injury
- Initiated/associated with a loud pop
- Isolated pain
- Unequal pain

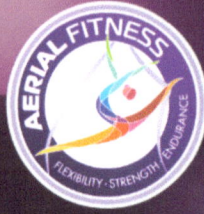

AERIAL FITNESS SUCCESS TIPS

1 EXERCISE DAILY

2 MAKE HEALTHY FOOD CHOICES

3 STAY MOTIVATED

4 GET ENOUGH SLEEP

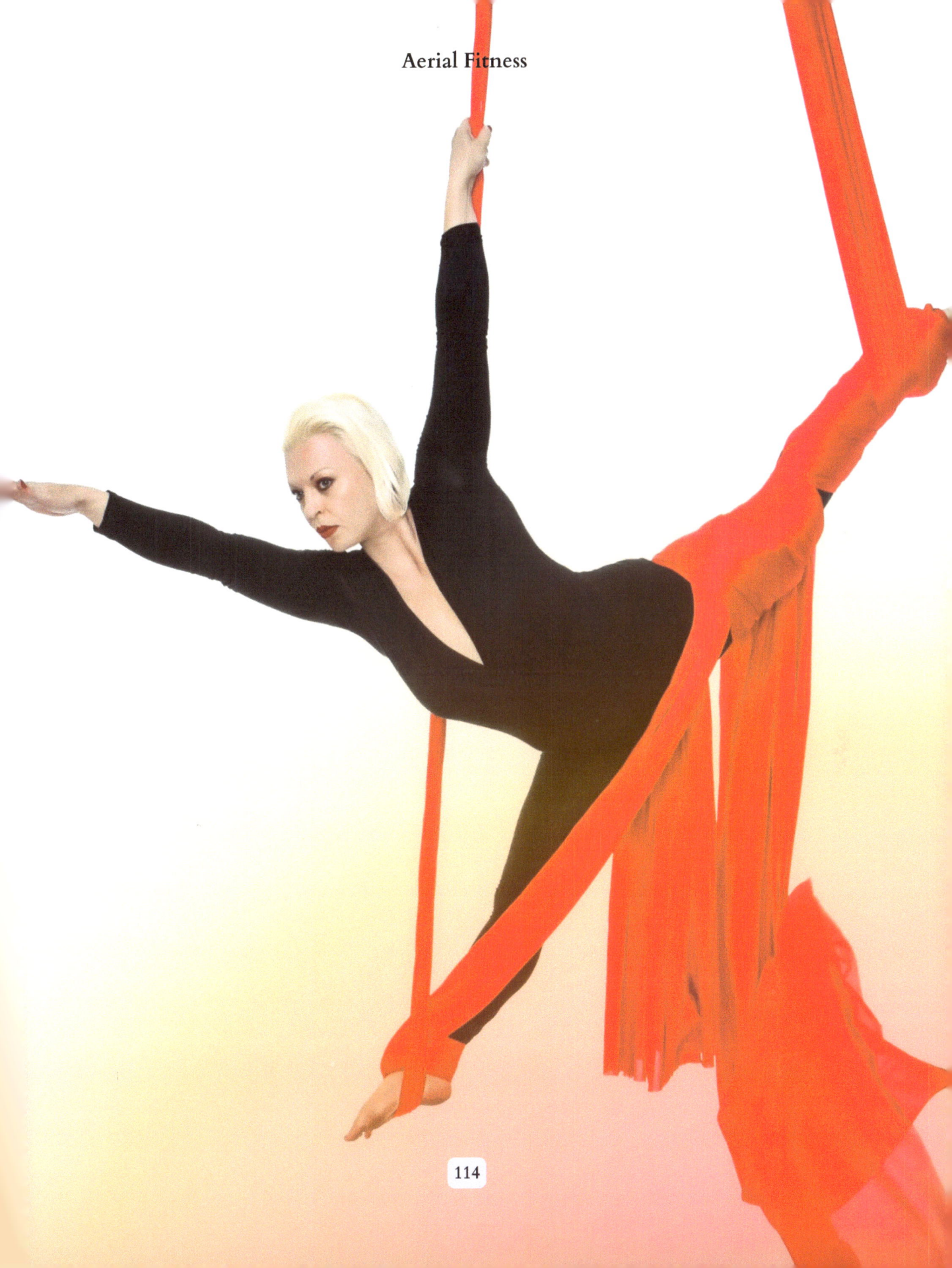

AERIAL FITNESS

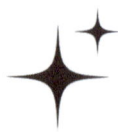

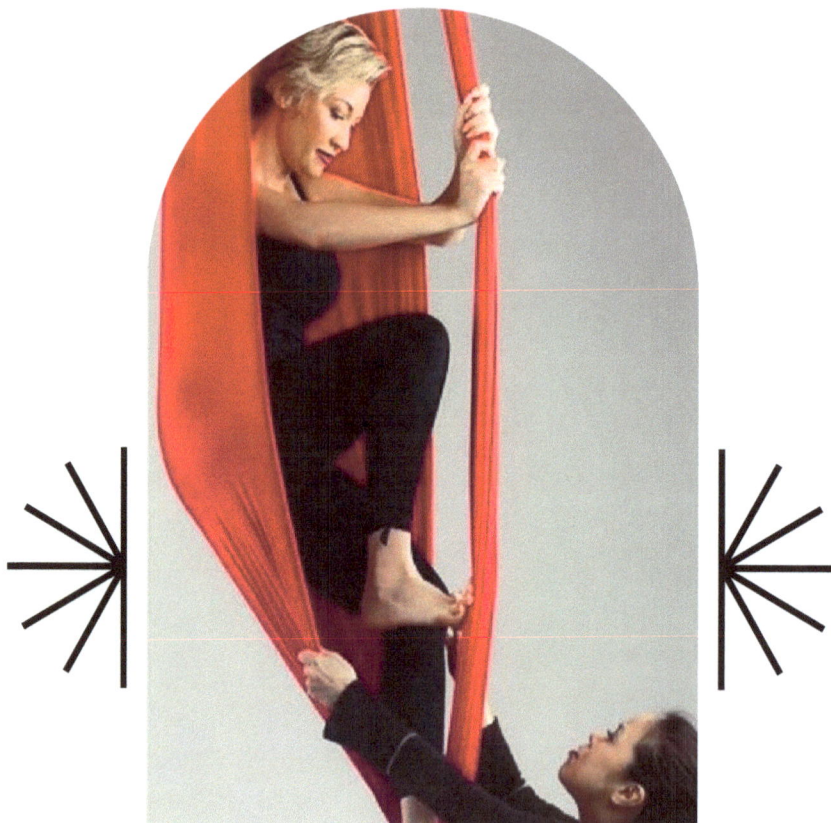

RESOURCES

EQUIPMENT & SUPPLIERS

U.S.A

AERIAL APPAREL
6040 S. FORT APACHE ROAD #101
LAS VEGAS, NV 89148
(702) 530-3031
INFO@AERIALAPPAREL.NET
WWW.AERIALAPPAREL.NET

AERIAL ESSENTIALS
4460 W. RENO AVENUE, SUITE G
LAS VEGAS, NV 89118
(702) 907-2359
WWW.AERIALESSENTIALS.COM

BLACK DIAMOND EQUIPMENT
(800) 775-5552
BDMO@BDEL.COM
WWW.BDEL.COM

BOBBY'S BIG TOP INC.
BOBBY BATES
(251) 979-1739
WWW.BOBBYSBIGTOP.COM

CIRCUS CONCEPTS
3527 BOUL INDUSTRIEL
SHERBROOKE, QUEBEC J1L 1X7
CANADA
(855) 203-5855
WWW.CIRCUSCONCEPTS.COM

CMI CORPORATION
338 MILL ROAD
PO BOX 535
FRANKLIN, WV 26807
(304) 358-7041
WWW.CMIGEARUSA.COM

CMC RESCUE
6740 CORTONA DRIVE
GOLETA, CA 93117
(800) 513-7455
INFO@CMCPRO.COM
WWW.CMCPRO.COM

CORDERIE CLÉMENT
11 RUE CHARLES MICHELS BP7
92222 BAGNEUX CEDEX
FRANCE
+33 01-45-36-12-34
WWW.CORDERIE-CLEMENT.FR

FIRE TOYS INC.
20 HAYPRESS ROAD, SUITE 311
CRANBURY, NJ, 08512
(844) 340-4580
CONTACT@FIRETOYS.COM
WWW.FIRETOYS.COM

FUSION TACTICAL
1680 S, GROVE AVENUE, SUITE #A
ONTARIO, CA 91761
(909) 393-9450
WWW.FUSIONTACTICALUSA.COM

KONG
VIA XXV APRILE, 4
23804 MONTE MARENZO (LC)
ITALY
+39 0341 630506
WWW.KONG.IT

OMEGA PACIFIC
11427 WEST 21ST AVENUE
AIRWAY HEIGHTS, WA 99001
(800) 360-3990
INFO@OMEGAPAC.COM
WWW.OMEGAPAC.COM

PETZL
(801) 926-1500
INFO@PETZL.COM
WWW.PETZL.COM

PMI
4466 N HWY 27
PO BOX 803
LAFAYETTE, GA 30728-0803
(706) 764-1437
CUSTSERV@PMIROPE.COM
WWW.PMIROPE.COM

EQUIPMENT & SUPPLIERS

REI
SUMNER, WA 98352-0001
(800) 426-4840
WWW.REI.COM

RENEGADE JUGGLING
727 ALMAR AVENUE
SANTA CRUZ, CA 95060
(831) 426-7343
WWW.RENEGADEJUGGLING.COM

ROCK EXOTICA
FREEPORT CENTER, BUILDING E-16
CLEARFIELD, UT 84016
(801) 728-0630
INFO@ROCKEXOTICA.COM
WWW.ROCKEXOTICA.COM

ROCK-N-RESCUE
300 DELWOOD ROAD
BUTLER, PA 16001
(724) 256-8822
WWW.ROCKNRESCUE.COM

SAPSIS RIGGING INC.
(800) 727-7471
SALES@SAPSIS-RIGGING.COM
WWW.SAPSIS-RIGGING.COM

SEATTLE MANUFACTURING COMPANY
930 SALASHAN PARKWAY
FERNDALE, WA 98248
(800) 426-6251
CUSTOMERSERVICE@SMCGEAR.COM
WWW.SMCGEAR.COM

TRAPEZE ARTS INC.
1822 9TH STREET
OAKLAND, CA 94607
(510) 419-0700
INFO@TRAPEZEARTS.COM
WWW.TRAPEZEARTS.COM

TRIX CIRCUS
+61 404 536 367
AUSTRALIA
INFO@TRIXCIRCUS.COM
WWW.TRIXCIRCUS.COM

X-POLE
12721 SATICOY STREET SOUTH
NORTH HOLLYWOOD, CA 91605
(818) 514-7325
INFO@XPOLEUS.COM
WWW.XPOLEUS.COM

RIGGING PROVIDERS

FOY INVENTERPRISES
3275 EAST PATRICK LANE
LAS VEGAS, NV 89120
USA
(702) 454-3500
WWW.FLYBYFOY.COM

FOY INVENTERPRISES EUROPE
UNIT 4, BOREHAMWOOD ENTERPRISE CENTRE
THEOBALD STREET
BOREHAMWOOD
HERTFORDSHIRE
WD6 4RQ, UK
+44 (0)20 8236 0234
WWW.FLYBYFOY.COM

VERTIGO
241 W. STEPHENIE DRIVE
CORTLAND, IL 60112
(888) 359-4255
INFO@GETVERTIGO.COM
WWW.GETVERTIGO.COM

ZFX FLYING INC.
611 INDUSTRY ROAD
LOUISVILLE, KY 40208
(502) 637-2500
WWW.ZFXFLYING.COM

STUDIO LISTINGS

ACTOR'S GYMNASIUM
927 NOYES STREET
EVANSTON, IL 60201
(847) 328-2795
EMAIL@ACTORSGYMNASIUM.ORG
WWW.ACTORSGYMNASIUM.ORG

AERIAL FITNESS
6040 S. FORT APACHE ROAD #101
LAS VEGAS, NV 89148
(702) 886-2250
INFO@AERIAL-FITNESS.NET
WWW.AERIAL-FITNESS.NET

AERIAL PHYSIQUE
4700 WEST JEFFERSON BLVD. SUITE 107
LOS ANGELES, CA 90016
(800) 208-2246
WWW.AERIALPHYSIQUE.COM

ALOFT
3324 W WRIGHTWOOD AVENUE
CHICAGO, IL 60647
(312) 771-2478
CHRISTINEALOFT@GMAIL.COM
WWW.ALOFTLOFT.COM

CANOPY STUDIO, INC.
160 TRACY STREET
ATHENS, GA 30601
(706) 549-8501
WWW.CANOPYSTUDIO.ORG

CHARLOTTE CIRQUE & DANCE CENTER
9315 MONROE ROAD
CHARLOTTE, NC 28270
(704) 844-0449
WWW.CAROLINECALOUCHE.ORG

CIRCADIUM
6452 GREENE STREET
PHILADELPHIA, PA 19119
(215) 849-1991
INFO@CIRCADIUM.COM
WWW.CIRCADIUM.COM

CIRCUS ARTS INSTITUTE, LLC
ATLANTA, GA
(404) 549-3000
WWW.CIRCUSARTSINSTITUTE.COM

CIRCUS HARMONY
701 N 15TH. STREET
SAINT LOUIS, MO 63103
(314) 436-7676
WWW.CIRCUSHARMONY.ORG

CIRCUS UP! % COMMONWEALTH CIRCUS CENTER
8 BROOKLEY ROAD
JAMAICA PLAIN, MA 02130
(617) 826-9487
WWW.CIRCUSUP.COM

CIRCUS WAREHOUSE
53-21 VERNON BOULEVARD
LONG ISLAND CITY, NY 11101
(212) 751-2174
INFO@CIRCUSWAREHOUSE.COM
WWW.CIRCUSWAREHOUSE.COM

CIRQUELOUIS
4648 GRAND DELL DRIVE
CRESTWOOD, KY 40014
(502) 509-8541
WWW.CIRQUELOUIS.COM

DIAMOND FAMILY CIRCUS
34 FRANCIS STREET
WALTHAM, MA 02451
WWW.DIAMONDCIRCUS.COM

ENCPR ESCUELA NACIONAL DE CIRCO DE PUERTO RICO
LAS FLORES 123
SAN JUAN, 00911
PUERTO RICO
(787) 678-7103
WWW.CIRCOPR.ORG

ESH CIRCUS ARTS
44 PARK STREET
SOMERVILLE, MA 02143
(617) 764-0190
INFO@ESHCIRCUSARTS.COM
WWW.ESHCIRCUSARTS.COM

STUDIO LISTINGS

FERN STREET CIRCUS
P.O. BOX 5864
SAN DIEGO, CA 92165
(619) 320-2055
WWW.FERNSTREETCIRCUS.COM

FREQUENT FLYERS AERIAL DANCE
3022 E. STERLING CIRCLE #150
BOULDER, CO 80301
(303) 245-8272
WWW.FREQUENTFLYERS.ORG

KINETIC THEORY
4723 EXPOSITION BOULEVARD
LOS ANGELES, CA 90016
(323) 402-0773
INFO@KINETICTHEORYTHEATRE.COM
WWW.KINETICTHEORYTHEATRE.COM

LE PETIT CIRQUE
8717 AVIATION BLVD.
INGLEWOOD, CA 90301
(310) 962-0737
WWW.LESTUDIOLA.COM/LE-PETIT-CIRQUE

MADISON CIRCUS SPACE
84 N. BRYAN STREET
MADISON, WI 53704
(608) 284-8744
WWW.MADISONCIRCUSSPACE.COM

MY NOSE TURNS RED
10500 READING ROAD
CINCINNATI, OH 44241
(859) 581-7100
WWW.MYNOSETURNSRED.ORG

NEW ENGLAND CENTER FOR CIRCUS ARTS
10 TOWN CRIER DRIVE
BRATTLEBORO VT 05301
(802) 254-9780
INFO@NECENTERFORCIRCUSARTS.ORG
WWW.NECENTERFORCIRCUSARTS.ORG

NEWBURGH COMMUNITY CIRCUS PROJECT
85 MINE HILL ROAD
CORNWALL, NY 12518
(845) 458-5414
WWW.SAFE-HARBOURS.ORG/?S=CIRCUS

PENASCO CIRCUS THEATRE
P.O. BOX 313
PEÑASCO, NM 87553
(575) 770-7597
WWW.PENASCOTHEATERCOLLECTIVE.ORG

SAMADHI HAWAII
330 COOKE STREET
HONOLULU, HI 96813
(808) 683-6080
WWW.SAMADHIHAWAII.COM

SAN DIEGO CIRCUS CENTER
2050 HANCOCK STREET, SUITE A
SAN DIEGO, CA 92110
(619) 487-1239
INFO@SANDIEGOCIRCUSCENTER.ORG
WWW.SANDIEGOCIRCUSCENTER.ORG

SAN FRANCISCO CIRCUS CENTER
755 FREDERICK STREET
SAN FRANCISCO, CA 94117
(415) 759-8123
INFO@CIRCUSCENTER.ORG
WWW.CIRCUSCENTER.ORG

SCHOOL OF ACROBATICS AND NEW CIRCUS ARTS
674 SOUTH ORCAS STREET
SEATTLE, WA 98108
(206) 652-4433
OFFICE@SANCASEATTLE.ORG
WWW.SANCASEATTLE.ORG

THE CIRCUS ACADEMY OF TUSCON
400 W. SPEEDWAY BLVD.
TUCSON, AZ 85705
(928) 814-9637
WWW.CIRCUSACADEMYTUCSON.COM

STUDIO LISTINGS

THE CIRCUS PROJECT
1420 NW 17TH AVENUE, SUITE 388
PORTLAND, OR 97209
(503) 764–9174
FRONTDESK@THECIRCUSPROJECT.ORG
WWW.THECIRCUSPROJECT.ORG

THE MUSE BROOKLYN
350 MOFFAT STREET
BROOKLYN, NY 11237
(929) 400–1678
WWW.THEMUSEBROOKLYN.COM

THE SELLAM CIRCUS SCHOOL
40 MAIN STREET, BLDG. 13, SUITE 135
BIDDEFORD, ME 04005
(207) 502-2589
INFO@THESELLAMCIRCUS.COM
WWW.THESELLAMCIRCUS.COM

VERSATILE ARTS
7601 GREENWOOD AVENUE NORTH
SEATTLE, WA 98103
(866) 887-5256
WWW.VERSATILEARTS.NET

THE VERTICAL FIX
7425 S HARL AVENUE
TEMPE, AZ 85283
(623) 850–8155
INFO@THEVERTICALFIX.COM
WWW.THEVERTICALFIX.COM

VERTIFIT AERIAL ARTS
880 AIRPORT ROAD
ORMOND BEACH, FL 32174
(516) 695-4077
WWW.VERTIFIT.COM

WISE FOOL NEW MEXICO
1131 SILER ROAD, SUITE B
SANTA FE, NM 87507
(505) 992-2588
WWW.WISEFOOLNEWMEXICO.ORG

AUSTRALIA

CIRCUS OZ
35 JOHNSTON STREET
COLLINGWOOD, VICTORIA 3066
+61 3 9676 0300
WWW.CIRCUSOZ.COM

CANADA

ATLANTIC CIRQUE LTD.
30 OLAND COURT
DARTMOUTH, NOVA SCOTIA
B3B 1V2
(902) 457-2227
ADMIN@ATLANTICCIRQUE.COM
WWW.ATLANTICCIRQUE-HALIFAX.COM/

CIRCUSWEST
2901 EAST HASTINGS STREET
VANCOUVER, BC
V5K 5J1
(604) 252-3679
WWW.CIRCUSWEST.COM

DYNAMIC AERIAL AND ACROBATICS
6039 196 STREET #109
SURREY, BRITISH COLUMBIA
(604) 539-2296
DYNAMICAERIALANDACROBATICS@GMAIL.COM
WWW.DYNAMICAERIALANDACROBATICS.COM

ÉCOLE NATIONALE DE CIRQUE
8181 AVENUE DU CIRQUE
MONTREAL, QUEBEC
CANADA H1Z 4N9
(514) 982-0859
TOLL FREE IN CANADA: (800) 267-0859
INFO@ENC.QC.CA
WWW.ECOLENATIONALEDECIRQUE.CA

STUDIO LISTINGS

ÉCOLE DE CIRQUE DE QUÉBEC
750, 2ND AVENUE
QUEBEC CITY, QUEBEC G1L 3B7
(418) 525-0101
INFO@ECOLEDECIRQUE.COM
WWW.ECOLEDECIRQUE.COM

LE CHÂTEAU DE CIRQUE
6956 ST-DENIS
MONTREAL, QUEBEC
(514) 251-0615
WWW.CHATEAU-CIRQUE.COM

THE CIRCUS LAB
#3 - 19840 96TH AVENUE
LANGLEY, BC
(604) 357 - 5277
INFO@THECIRCUSLAB.CA
WWW.THECIRCUSLAB.CA

TORONTO SCHOOL OF CIRCUS ARTS
75 CARL HALL ROAD, UNIT 8
PARC DOWNSVIEW PARK, M3K 2B9
(416) 935-0037
WWW.TORONTOCIRCUS.COM

VANCOUVER CIRCUS SCHOOL
810 QUAYSIDE DRIVE
NEW WESTMINSTER, BC V3M 6B9
(604) 544-5024
INFO@VANCOUVERCIRCUSSCHOOL.CA
WWW.VANCOUVERCIRCUSCHOOL.CA

ENGLAND

CIRCOMEDIA
ST PAUL'S CHURCH
PORTLAND SQUARE
BRISTOL, BS2 8SJ
+44 0117 924 7615
INFO@CIRCOMEDIA.COM
WWW.CIRCOMEDIA.COM

NATIONAL CENTRE FOR CIRCUS ARTS
CORONET STREET
LONDON
N1 6HD
+44 020 7613 4141
INFO@NATIONALCIRCUS.ORG.UK
WWW.NATIONALCIRCUS.ORG.UK

SINGAPORE

AERIAL FITNESS STUDIO
LOCATED IN: ELTOV SINGAPORE
CT HUB 2 #01-42
114 LAVENDER STREET
SINGAPORE 338729
CONTACT@AERIALFITNESS.SG
WWW.AERIALFITNESS.SG

RIGGING INFORMATION

WWW.ANIMATEDKNOTS.COM

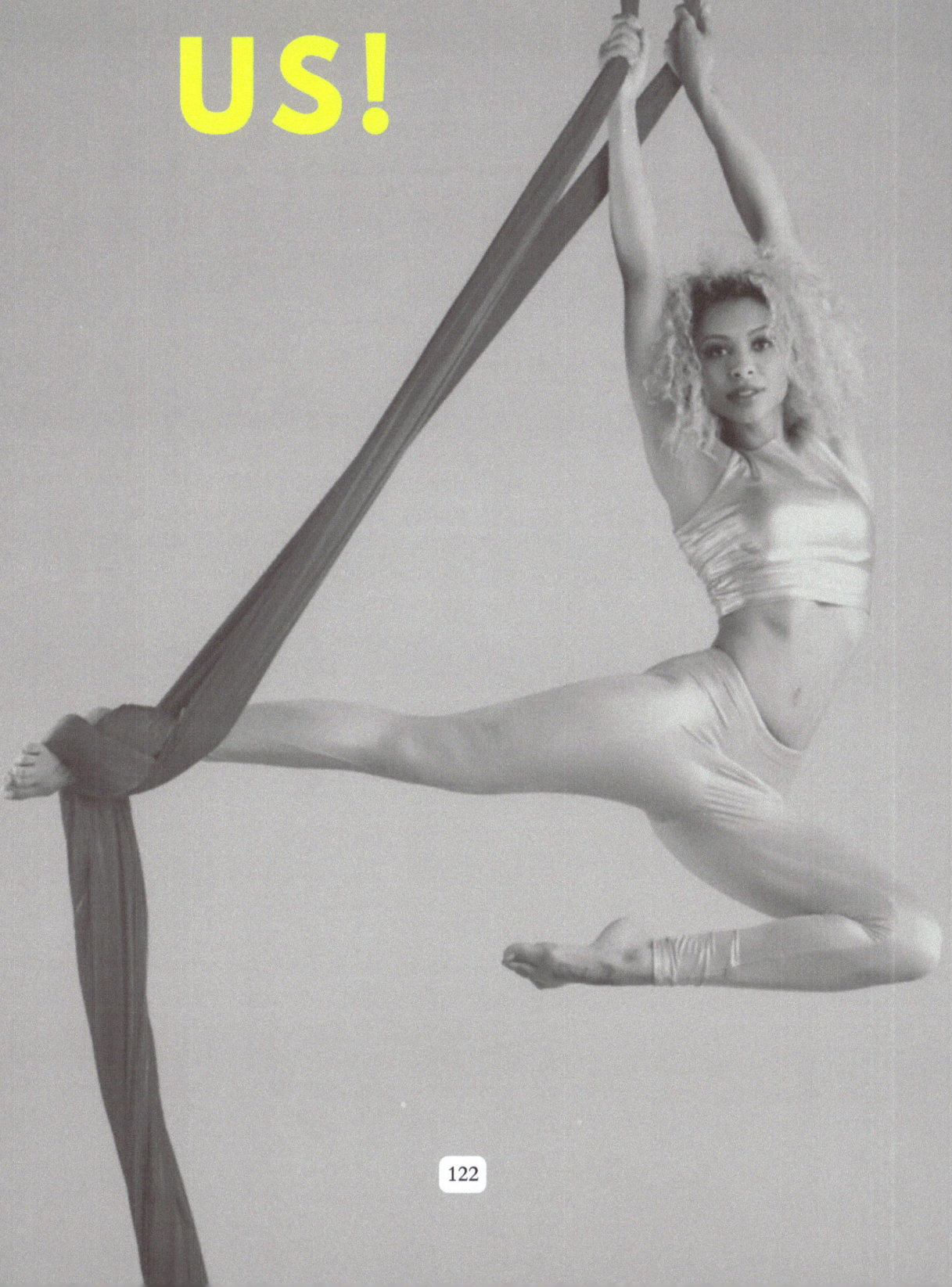

FLY WITH US!

AERIAL FITNESS INSTRUCTOR CERTIFICATION PROGRAM

Discover the art of Aerial Silks!

The Aerial Fitness Instructor Certification Program was designed to help you become a safe, knowledgeable, and skilled Aerial Fitness instructor. This course focuses on building a solid foundation of technique while learning how to adapt your teaching style to cater to each individual student.

Aerial Fitness Studio in Las Vegas, Nevada, provides training in Kristi Toguchi's Aerial Fitness, aerial acrobatics, flexibility, dance, contortion, performance, and magic. Kristi Toguchi's Aerial Fitness program will focus on building your core strength and flexibility as you learn exercises moving your body on both the ground and the air. Aerial Fitness classes are full-body workouts that will emphasize building technique and proper alignment. You will learn the basic skills and techniques that will help you achieve your fitness goals.

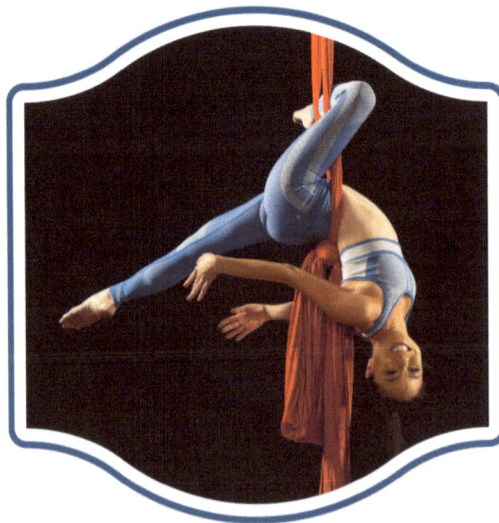

FOR MORE INFORMATION VISIT
www.AerialFitnessCertification.com

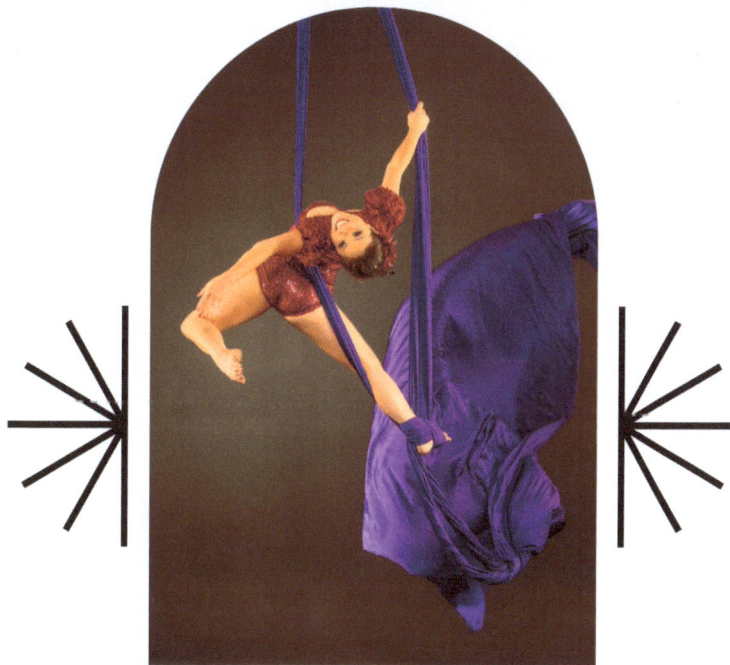

YEARLY GOALS

January

February

March

April

May

June

July

August

September

October

November

December

125

Month: Week:

Aerial Fitness Planner

WARM-UP

CONDITIONING
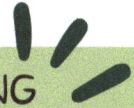

AERIAL SKILLS

COMBINATION
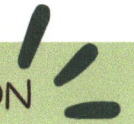

Month: Week:

Aerial Fitness Planner

WARM-UP

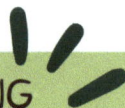

CONDITIONING

AERIAL SKILLS

COMBINATION

127

Aerial Fitness

Plan

EXERCISE ROUTINE 01

NOTES

○ ....

○ ....

○ ....

EXERCISE ROUTINE 02

○ ....

○ ....

○ ....

EXERCISE ROUTINE 03

○ ....

○ ....

○ ....

Aerial Fitness Plan

EXERCISE ROUTINE 01

NOTES

○ ....

○ ....

○ ....

EXERCISE ROUTINE 02

○ ....

○ ....

○ ....

EXERCISE ROUTINE 03

○ ....

○ ....

○ ....

AERIAL FITNESS PLANNER

s	m	t	w	t	f	s	Exercise

Warm-Up & Cool-Down

Combination

Notes

AERIAL FITNESS PLANNER

s	m	t	w	t	f	s	Exercise

Warm-Up & Cool-Down

Combination

Notes

YEARLY GOALS

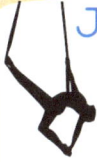

January

February

March

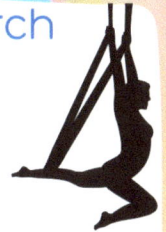

April

May

June

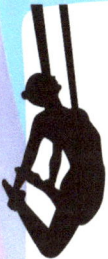

July

August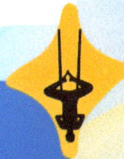

September

October

November

December

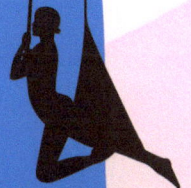

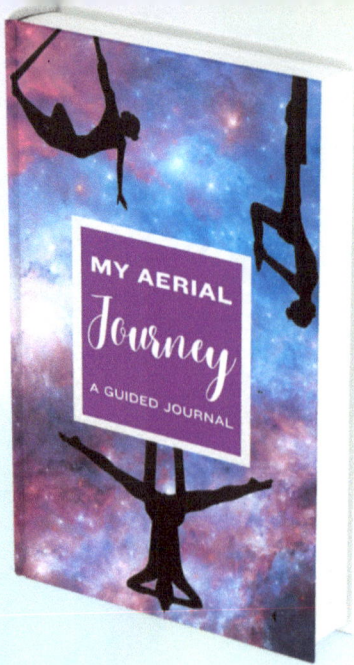

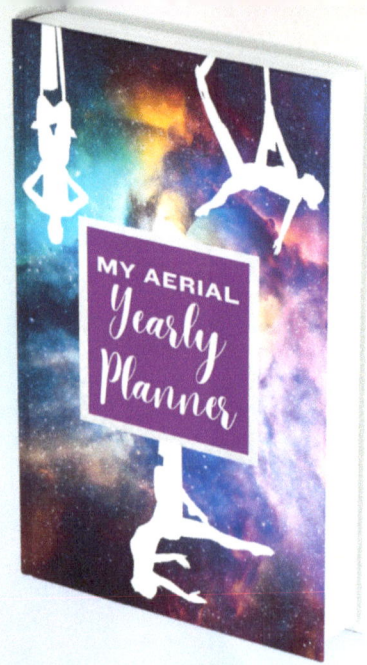

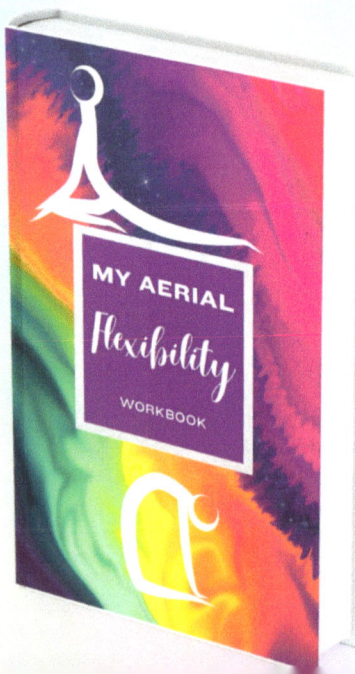

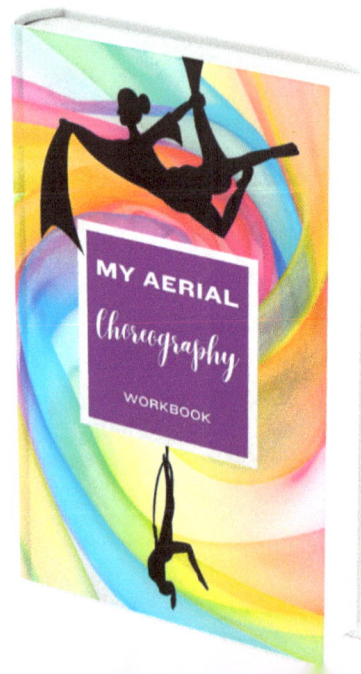

133

STAY CONNECTED

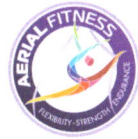

AERIAL FITNESS LLC

Kristi Toguchi

(702) 886-2250

www.AerialFitness.us

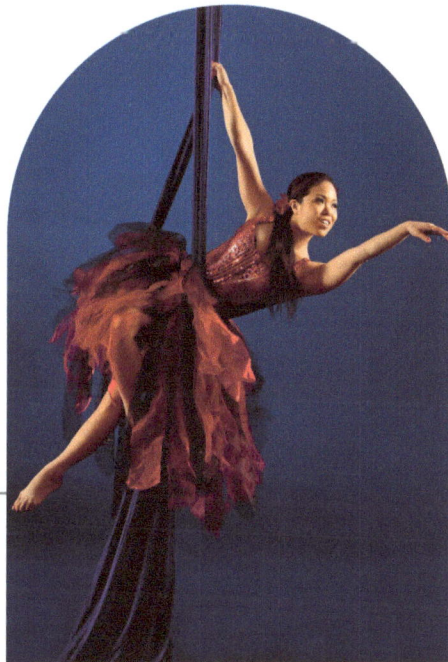

www.ingramcontent.com/pod-product-compliance
Lightning Source LLC
Chambersburg PA
CBHW060900270326
41935CB00004B/51